Conversing with Cancer

Language as SOCIAL ACTION

Howard Giles
General Editor

Vol. 22

The Language as Social Action series
is part of the Peter Lang Media and Communication list.
Every volume is peer reviewed and meets
the highest quality standards for content and production.

PETER LANG
New York • Bern • Berlin
Brussels • Vienna • Oxford • Warsaw

Lisa Sparks and Anna Leahy

Conversing with Cancer

How to Ask Questions, Find and Share Information, and Make the Best Decisions

PETER LANG
New York • Bern • Berlin
Brussels • Vienna • Oxford • Warsaw

Library of Congress Cataloging-in-Publication Data

Names: Sparks, Lisa, author. | Leahy, Anna, author.
Title: Conversing with cancer: how to ask questions, find and share information, and make the best decisions / Lisa Sparks and Anna Leahy.
Description: New York: Peter Lang, 2018.
Series: Language as social action; vol. 22 | ISSN 1529-2436
Includes bibliographical references and index.
Identifiers: LCCN 2017030332 | ISBN 978-1-4331-3354-1 (hardback: alk. paper)
ISBN 978-1-4331-3353-4 (paperback: alk. paper) | ISBN 978-1-4331-3900-0 (ebook pdf)
ISBN 978-1-4331-3901-7 (epub) | ISBN 978-1-4331-3902-4 (mobi)
Subjects: LCSH: Cancer—Social aspects.
Cancer—Psychological aspects.
Communication in medicine.
Classification: LCC RC262 .S64 | DDC 362.19699/4—dc23
LC record available at https://lccn.loc.gov/2017030332
DOI 10.3726/b13076

Bibliographic information published by **Die Deutsche Nationalbibliothek.**
Die Deutsche Nationalbibliothek lists this publication in the "Deutsche Nationalbibliografie"; detailed bibliographic data are available on the Internet at http://dnb.d-nb.de/.

29 Broadway, 18th floor, New York, NY 10006
www.peterlang.com

We dedicate *Conversing with Cancer* to our families and friends, past, present, and future, including Daniele, Alessandro, Elena, Arianna, Athena, and parents John O. and Marcia and Douglas, Brigid, Maggie, and parents Andrew and Mary Lee.

TABLE OF CONTENTS

ACKNOWLEDGMENTS

We extend sincere thanks and acknowledgement to Howie Giles, a strong mentor in the field of communication. We also acknowledge the many at Peter Lang for making this book and the Language as Social Action series happen. We are truly grateful for this opportunity to contribute to the ongoing conversation about health communication and cancer care and to make a difference in the lives of patients and their families.

Sincere thanks to Chapman University undergraduate students Shoshanna Feld-Sobol and Brooke Grogan. Also, thanks to graduate students Mike Gravagno, Samantha Mountjoy, Mackenzie Bates, Alysia Hendry, and Devin Valasco for the many ways they helped shape this book, especially the penultimate chapter and the glossary. Also, thanks to Mary Cantrell, Brigid Leahy, Paulette Livers, and Patricia Grace King for their editorial acumen and suggestions as we drafted early chapters. Finally, to those many individuals who have written about their experiences in their own books and blogs and, in some cases, in personal exchanges with us, we are grateful to be able to talk about their stories in *Conversing with Cancer*.

Each chapter begins with an epigraph drawn from a poem. We thank the authors for their permission (with all rights reserved) to include an excerpt or whole poem, as space and topic allowed:

"at the doctor's" by Ivy Alvarez, *Mortal.* Washington, DC: Red Morning Press, 2006. Reprinted by permission of the author.

"Triolet on Beating the Odds" by permission of author Lanette Cadle.

"Exoskeleton" by Risa Denenberg, *Mean Distance from the Sun*, Aldrich Press, 2013. Reprinted by permission of the author.

"Chemo Room" by permission of author Penny Harter.

"Diagnosis" by permission of author Karen Paul Holmes.

"Google Moon (2)" by permission of author Anna Leahy.

"The Habits of Light" by Anna Leahy, *Aperture*, Shearsman Books, 2017. Reprinted by permission of the author.

"In the ICU" by Lesléa Newman, *I Carry My Mother*, Headmistress Press, 2015. Reprinted by permission of the author.

"Biopsy" by permission of author Stacy Nigliazzo.

"Cancer Diagnosis" by permission of author Marjorie Maddox and translator Rei Berroa; italics from *Hamlet*, Act I, Scene 2, lines 133–134. The English original appeared in *Fine Frenzy: Poets Respond to Shakespeare*, University of Iowa Press, and *Local News from Someplace Else*, Wipf and Stock Publishers. The Spanish translation appeared in *Luna Luna*.

"The Music Box" by Frank L. Meyskens Jr., *Believing in Today*, Fithian Press, 2014. Reprinted by permission of the publisher.

"Something Understood by permission of author Anya Silver.

In addition, excerpts from the blog of Patricia Grace King and from the Caring Bridge journal of Adam Schmitz were used as chapter epigraphs and discussed in the text. Patricia Grace King and Wooten Lee Schmitz graciously gave permission for use of these excerpts.

· 1 ·

INTRODUCTION TO *CONVERSING WITH CANCER*

When you feel something not-neck in your neck,
you can't possibly think *breast*

and don't realize that the Latin for *neck*
is *cervix*, that shape is one kind of connection,

that *metastasis* means *transition* or *removal* or
going somewhere else. And you want to be elsewhere

or you want to be here but otherwise,
and that doesn't mean you don't know the odds.

When I Google the Moon, it looks like
a milky mammogram: dense cells implied

by lunar crust, basalt-limned, marred and pocked,
cirrus threads connect maria and duct.

Cognitum is the sea that has become known,
but you don't feel you're drowning.

Marginis is the sea with irregular edges.
Nectaris is the sweet, dark ocean of long ago.

You follow the physician
into the phone booth and, for a moment, forever,

go somewhere—some other time—in the universe.
You're not lost here, in your lake of dreams.
—"Google Moon (2)" by Anna Leahy

Why You Need to Read This Book

With more than 40% of people eventually facing a cancer diagnosis, *Conversing with Cancer* is a much-needed addition to understanding and improving cancer care through strong communication among providers, patients, and caregivers. Each person whose life is affected by a cancer diagnosis—patient, healthcare provider, caregiver—has information and needs information in order to make the best decisions possible under the circumstances. After studying and writing about the topics of communication and cancer for many years separately, authors Lisa Sparks and Anna Leahy combine their expertise in this new tour de force. Here, they apply principles from the field of health communication to the cancer care experience, drawing from a wide range of scholarship to offer a comprehensive view of cancer care communication and extend existing work into new insights. Engaging chapters cover all phases of the cancer care continuum, from prevention to recovery or end-of-life; analyze the roles of the variety of cultural and social identities and relationships; and explore written, verbal, non-verbal, and electronic communication. In addition, this book draws from the real-life stories of cancer patients themselves to enrich the book's unique discussions and to better understand how theory can be put into practice. *Conversing with Cancer* is ideal for use in health communication classes, medical and nursing programs, and formal caregiver training. In addition, it is useful for cancer patient and caregiver supports groups and for individual providers, patients, and caregivers.

Each person whose life is affected by a cancer diagnosis—patient, healthcare provider, caregiver—has information and needs information in order to make the best decisions possible under the circumstances. Other books, brochures, and websites contain a wealth of biomedical information about specific cancer types, but few discuss at length how to acquire, sort, share, and use information to make the best healthcare decisions in difficult and complex situations. Within the field of communication, language use, messaging, and other communicative acts are understood both as manifestations of the social reality and as means for shaping the social reality. Scholars of health communication apply this understanding and the scholarly approaches of the field in an effort to create shared meaning about health care and conditions. This book draws from a variety of theoretical and evidence-based approaches to analyze communication within the context of the continuum of cancer care, with particular attention to real-life scenarios documented by patients, caregivers, and providers.

Once diagnosed with cancer, a person may feel as if he or she is always *with* cancer, that every conversation, thought, or action is altered by this new state of being as a cancer patient (Sparks, 2003, 2013). Especially at first, the patient may feel as if *healthcare providers*—those people authorized to deliver medical and health services, including physicians—are speaking a kind of gibberish filled with Latin names for the disease, using shorthand for symptoms, and tossing around acronyms for chemotherapy combinations. The patient and the patient's family may be sorting through what cancer staging and tumor marker levels mean for decisions about treatment and for their day-to-day lives. They may struggle to disentangle risks, benefits, and side effects of different treatments and figure out which pros and cons are most important to their decisions about the next steps and their own lives as well as which benefits and risks the oncologist emphasizes. Often, the patient or family member may not know how to put fears and confusions into words and may not know what kinds of questions will get the answers that are most needed. From our own experiences as caregivers, we know that a deeper knowledge of communication processes helps a person negotiate this difficult time, offers ways to exert some control in a sometimes overwhelming situation, and leads to better health outcomes for the individual.

Scholars in health communication recognize that information about type and stage of cancer and treatment options is like a list of ingredients in a recipe for a meal they've never had before. The ingredients are necessary to have, of course, but without instructions for what to do with them, the patient and caregivers may still feel lost as to how to move from one step to the next. Communication helps an individual put the ingredients together—whether to stir or to blend, which substitutions can be made without messing up the result, what temperature works best, and how to tell when enough is enough. Many patients, providers, and caregivers may not realize they can improve healthcare communication among each other and may not realize how much that improvement can matter to a patient's sense of well-being and one's healthcare outcomes. *Conversing with Cancer*—the book and the website Cancer Culture Communication (www.conversingwithcancer.com)—can guide health communication scholars and students as well as patients, caregivers, and healthcare providers.

Why We Wrote This Book

As the authors of *Conversing with Cancer*, we have been studying this topic for more than twenty-five years combined. We have made our own individual contributions to literature about cancer and communication, and now we have come together to share what we have learned through research, reading, and experience. *Conversing with Cancer* draws from numerous health communication scholars with whom Lisa Sparks has collaborated and also creative writers whose work Anna Leahy has analyzed. Importantly, we draw from our own caregiving experiences too.

Health communication is the study of how information about health and health care is and can be communicated, whether through public health campaigns, individual or community health literacy and education, or provider–patient conversations about a specific situation. Sparks (2013) defines health communication as the following: "health communication *involves creating shared meaning about health care and conditions*" (p. 132). Health communication covers a wide-range of topics, including disease control and prevention, emergency preparedness and response, injury and violence prevention, environmental health, workplace safety, and general communication behavior as it relates to well-being and leading healthy lives. On the national level, efforts to promote health often use a developmental-life-span perspective and a focus on age (e.g., adolescent health, health among the aging), gender (e.g., women's health issues such as family planning, men's health issues such as testicular cancer), community health (e.g., school health and nonprofits), and health among particular minorities (Parrott, 2004; Sparks & Villagran, 2008, 2010). Health communication as a field is thriving, with important applications to many health contexts, particularly in areas of cancer communication as well as contributions to related research, policy, and practice.

The approach that the field of health communication takes echoes the approaches of some other fields, such as anthropology and sociology. S. Lochlann Jain (2013) is an anthropologist, and the way she defines *cancer* in the introduction of her book *Malignant* is useful: "Anything *but* an objective thing, cancer can be better understood as a set of relationships—economic, sentimental, medical, personal, ethical, institutional, statistical" (p. 4). Health communication and *Conversing with Cancer*, however, focus on the set of relationships among individuals and other entities that have and share information about health and health care. The health communication research that informs this book makes it a reliable, useful guide for our readers. The information we draw together acknowledges cancer as a biomedical situation that requires medical treatment and also as a complicated social, interpersonal, and sociocultural situation that involves a range of communication issues in individual lives. As authors of this book, it is our sincere hope and goal that all involved in cancer care—scholars, students, patients, caregivers, healthcare providers, researchers—have access to this crucial information about how best to communicate across the continuum of cancer care from prevention, detection, diagnosis, treatment, and survivorship, thriving, and/or end-of-life.

This book also uniquely draws from the experiences of real people who have written about their own cancer treatment in books and on blogs. These voices and stories make this book a rich, personal experience for our readers. Most importantly, we have been there as caregivers for our family members when they were diagnosed with cancer, so we know how difficult it can be to navigate the landscape once cancer looms as an obstacle in the path a person has set for one's life. We wrote *Conversing with Cancer* because we have a sincere and committed personal stake in improving health communication and cancer care for real people.

Why Health Communication Matters, or Why Status Quo Isn't Good Enough

Interaction matters. Back-and-forth exchanges count. What we say (and don't say), when and where we say it, how we reveal or elicit information, and why we say what we say—all these aspects of communication influence the decisions we make and the actions we take in relation to our health (e.g., Sparks, 2013, 2014; Sparks & Villagran, 2010; Wright, Sparks, & O'Hair, 2013). While that sounds like common sense, it is surprising how easily healthcare providers, patients, and caregivers overlook communication when faced with a crisis or unfamiliar terrain. We tend to muddle through.

Or worse. When information isn't shared, problems emerge. When information is not well understood or is not used to make better decisions, problems can occur (Kreps & Sparks, 2015; Sparks, 2013, 2014). Physicians, for instance, know how germs are transmitted. They have learned about germs and how some infections can be transmitted in human-to-human contact, and patients depend on physicians to apply that knowledge in their work. That is precisely why doctors wash their hands between patients. Research several years ago, however, showed that the neckties many male physicians wear carry germs and that doctors often adjust their neckties with the hands they also use to examine patients (Day, 2006). We assumed, then, that doctors would have stopped wearing neckties immediately, and, in fact, we knew some physicians happy to ditch them and other physicians who were not wearing them in the first place. So, why, years later in 2014, did the Society for Healthcare Epidemiology of America have to issue new guidelines about healthcare provider attire in the journal *Infection Control and Hospital Epidemiology* that addressed this necktie problem (Bearman et al., 2014). Either, the earlier research was not shared widely with healthcare professionals, or the information was not well understood or not properly used by healthcare organizations and physicians to make better decisions. Communication failed and put patients at risk of infection.

This new research, which reiterated the earlier study's findings, prompted new guidelines that might have been put into place after the earlier study. In this new study, one-third of physicians' neckties carried Staphylococcus aureus bacteria, and up to 70% of physicians admitted to *never* cleaning their neckties. This new study indicated that lab coats are germ carriers too, which makes sense. Think about that the next time a doctor tucks his tie into his lab coat as he leans over to palpate your body. While no one has claimed a direct link between neckties or lab coats and transmission of a specific infection to a specific patient, doctors should have enough common sense, even without professional fashion guidelines, to ditch neckties and launder lab coats more than once every twelve days, as the study indicated was common. Reporting research findings widely and publishing new guidelines that apply those findings are attempts to improve communication of information and, in turn, improve health care because common sense fell short. This example shows how the status quo may not be good enough and how communication can improve health care.

Lab coats also present other communication issues because they act as a cue during interpersonal exchanges. Not only do we need improved communication *about* lab coats and the potential for germ transmission, but lab coats also *are* a form of communication. Patients tend to like seeing doctors in white coats, in part because lab coats subtly communicate a comforting authority. This assumption about authority goes back at least to the research conducted by Stanley Milgram (1963). However, that authority may make it difficult for patients to question, contradict, or confront a physician even if that patient harbors questions or concerns. Both common sense and clear, open communication sometimes get put inadvertently aside by both healthcare providers and by patients. *Conversing with Cancer* tackles head on issues raised by these communicative examples. This book unpacks numerous and varied communication issues related to health care in the effort to increase shared meaning among each patient and the team of providers at each phase, each decision, and each pressure point involved in the cancer care journey.

When healthcare providers, patients, caregivers, and even researchers do not communicate effectively, mistakes can occur in cancer care. Scholars within the fields of medicine, nursing, and communication have extensively studied provider–patient communication over the last several decades, and the research consistently shows that how providers and patients communicate in healthcare settings can greatly impact an array of problems, including medical errors and malpractice suits as well as physical and psychological health outcomes (Sparks & Villagran, 2008, 2010; Wright et al., 2013). Further, an important Joint Commission (2012) report revealed that more than 80% of medical errors are due to communication breakdowns, especially when multiple healthcare providers are involved in a patient's care (see e.g., Sparks, 2013; Sparks & Nussbaum, 2008).

Sometimes a person thinks one is making a good decision even when that patient and the provider have not communicated clearly and openly enough. When not enough information is communicated back and forth, an individual—patient or provider—may fill in gaps with assumptions. If the patient harbors unspoken concerns about symptoms or treatment, for instance, the physician may be missing valuable information that would change the treatment options or affect other decisions about that patient's care (Sparks, 2013, 2014).

Research by Juanjuan Zhang explores why people in need of kidney transplants often turn down available kidneys, for instance. The vast majority of offers of a new kidney are refused, and most refusals occur because the kidney available is not a good match. Nine out of ten people refuse the kidney because that's the sound medical decision. That is good news. Misguided inferences, however, "lead one in ten people who refuse a kidney to do so in error," according to Zhang (2010). Ten percent of patients offered a good match say, *No*. Why would anyone turn down a good kidney that he or she needs?

In his book *Contagious*, which discusses how we make decisions about our behavior, Jonah Berger (2013, pp. 129–130) writes of the situation this way:

> Say you are the one hundredth person on the list. A kidney would have first been offered to the first person on the list, then the second, and so on. So to finally reach you, it must have been turned down by ninety-nine other people. [...] If so many others have refused this kidney, people assume it must not be very good. They infer it is low quality and are more likely to turn it down. [...] Thousands of patients turn down kidneys they should have accepted.

It is unlikely these patients communicated their inferences clearly to their treating physicians, and the treating physicians probably did not realize that patients were factoring mistaken beliefs into their decision-making. The physicians and patients did not share enough information for these patients to make the best decision.

Unfortunately, this kind of miscommunication can and does occur in cancer care. Consider how many decisions an oncologist and a cancer patient must make in the course of care. When information exists but is not communicated back and forth, that information is not as useful as it can be. Think about how better back-and-forth communication of information might allow cancer patients to ask for more information they can use, share inferences or assumptions they have, sort through and prioritize information to figure out what is most relevant to them, and become empowered in the important decisions about their own care. Open, clear, effective, two-way verbal and nonverbal communication between healthcare providers and patients can help people make better decisions for living the best life possible.

Health communication is education and empowerment through effective, evidence-based messaging and exchange. *Conversing with Cancer* can help improve healthcare communication that matters. Better communication of information and priorities can improve both provider and patient decision-making and cancer care.

Communication, Crisis, and Cancer

Clear, open communication is often difficult in the best of circumstances. A cancer diagnosis often throws a person and one's family into crisis mode (Sparks, 2003). One's focus changes instantly. One is presented with information and choices to make. The ability to access and sort through information in a crisis can be crucial. All that, however, may make communication more difficult than usual.

Think of it this way. On a clear day, an experienced private pilot, who has studied and practiced flying for a long time, navigates her small aircraft without consciously thinking about the decisions she is making to keep the plane aloft and heading where she wants to go. But when she finds herself suddenly in bad weather and surrounded by clouds, she must pay greater attention to what she's doing and why. With several tasks to keep track of at once and unable to see the landscape below, she becomes disoriented. Worse, even though she knows from her training that she should prioritize the information that the aircraft's instruments provide about how far above the ground the plane is and which end is up, her physical senses are telling her something else. Her whole body, upon which she has relied all her life, feels upside-down, even though the instrument panel tells her that she should not change the plane's course. If she is in range of an airport with air traffic control, they can tell her the plane's altitude, speed, and trajectory, which will help, but they won't know whether the plane is upside-down. She is missing the usual visual cues because the clouds are too thick. Within minutes, despite her previous experience flying, she really does not know whether to trust herself or the aircraft. The choice she must make between sets of information could mean life or death for that pilot.

A cancer diagnosis is like flying through a bad storm. In the context of cancer care, lack of clear, honest, and prioritized communication of a variety of information among provider, patient, and caregiver can lead unnecessarily to missed opportunities, tragic mistakes, and compromised quality of life. The physician can provide the patient information about cancer markers in the blood, for instance, but cancer markers may be an instrument the patient does not fully understand. The physician may not realize that the patient feels upside-down.

Luckily, the cancer patient has more time to sort through information than the pilot does. Both healthcare providers and patients can improve communication in a timely way. Cancer care is a special kind of health care especially amenable to improving communication through mutual effort of providers, patients, and caregivers. Someone in the emergency room (ER) with symptoms of a heart attack sees a doctor immediately and often is aggressively treated within minutes, even before a thorough diagnosis has been made or explained to the patient or family. Cancer care, however, allows some time to sort through a diagnosis and related options for treatment. Even a cancer patient (often with the aid of a family member) in crisis mode after a diagnosis can use communication to get information, establish priorities, and make the best decisions.

Pilots go through a lot of training for worst-case scenarios during flight. The cancer patient, on the other hand, often has little knowledge about cancer prior to a diagnosis. Fortunately, that patient is likely to be very involved in receiving, giving, and using information in decisions about treatment. While a cancer diagnosis can create a crisis in one's life, strong provider–patient communication can be learned as one goes along the care journey and can play an important, positive role through the entire process of cancer care.

The cancer patient may find oneself upside-down with many decisions to make about how to keep oneself oriented in one's own life, even if that means learning to fly upside-down sometimes. Many patients have been muddling through without effective communication for too long. Providers often have been struggling to find productive ways to talk with their patients, and patients may sometimes feel overwhelming emotions that make it difficult to communicate as effectively as they usually do. Many healthcare providers and patients have been depending on common sense, instead of working toward more open and clear communication. Common sense—and the status quo—can be riddled with mistaken assumptions or assumptions not appropriate for the situation. Strong communication addresses the problems of the status quo.

The balance between quantity of life and quality of life is one of the most important and most difficult areas for communication and decision-making in cancer care. If an oncologist lays out standard treatment options but does not make a *prognosis*—the likely or usual course of the disease—at least somewhat clear, a patient with an excellent chance of survival may assume that cancer equals death. That negative attitude could affect day-to-day quality of life as well as choices about treatment. In another situation, a patient may not think to ask about hospice or end-of-life care, which may lead a physician to assume that extending that patient's life is their shared priority, no matter the physical, emotional, or financial cost. Patients, of course, do not want to invite bad news, and many of us struggle to talk about our own *mortality*—the fact that we will eventually die—even when we are healthy. Still, a patient can signal the physician to offer information relevant to the patient's situation, and physicians can encourage open exchange as well. Health communication research and best practices that emerge from that research help guide that exchange toward creating shared meaning among all involved from the team of providers to the patient as well as family and loved ones.

The medical establishment has only recently begun to recognize the value of effective communication in relationships between patient and provider and of the connection between communication and health outcomes. All of us can do better conversing about and in the presence of cancer, and that is precisely why we wrote this book.

How This Book Can Improve Cancer Care

Conversing with Cancer is designed to educate health communication specialists and to strengthen communication among patients, formal healthcare providers, and informal providers, including family caregivers, so that individuals can work together to improve cancer care. We chose this title because *conversing* means *to turn together*, as when a farmer in days of yore found himself at the end of the row he was planting and guided his ox and plow to the next row to keep going. A cancer diagnosis is often unexpected and unwanted, but when the patient, treating physician, other healthcare professionals, informal caregivers, and family members communicate well, this team of individuals can better understand the numerous obstacles that cancer presents in a person's life. Together, they can make the turns needed to navigate a new direction in life and keep going.

Conversing with Cancer strives to help patients, providers, and caregivers negotiate cancer care with a bit less stress and greater comfort and control over the long haul. This book offers guidance to health communication scholars and students as they strive to improve communicative interaction in the cancer care continuum. Each reader will come to *Conversing with Cancer* for one's own different reasons.

The Language as Social Action series in which *Conversing with Cancer* is situated explores the ways in which language embodies social reality, and that is the approach this book takes at every step. This book will be particularly useful to researchers in health communication who seek to better understand how language is produced, received, and analyzed in the context of cancer. While all chapters explore aspects of language as social reality and social action, Chapter 11 may be the most important for the academic scholar seeking to extend current research.

In addition to addressing academics in the field of communication studies, this book is designed for students, who may embark on academic research of their own, go on to work in healthcare organizations, or be in positions to shape social policy in the future. Students in health communication—junior scholars, so to speak—will gain a comprehensive understanding of how classroom concepts apply to real lives affected by cancer. By addressing students in addition to practicing scholars in communication studies, this book's principles can have long-term positive effects in the healthcare system and in communities.

Conversing with Cancer is also meant to be useful to the healthcare provider. You may be a physician, perhaps an oncologist who treats patients with cancer every day, a surgeon who has to report good and bad news about tumor excision, a general practitioner who sees patients over a lifetime, or perhaps you suddenly find yourself in the important informal role as a family caregiver. You may be a physician who is more adept at reading CT scans than listening to the person whose body you are viewing. Maybe one of your patients has recommended this book to you—we hope that patients who read this book will encourage their healthcare providers to read it. Nurses, medical technicians, healthcare administrators, social workers, hospice caregivers, and family caregivers will learn a great deal from this book about how to form productive partnerships with cancer patients, whether you see that patient once or over the course of treatment.

Of course, patients are at the center of the social reality of the continuum of cancer care. Perhaps, you have picked up this book because you have been diagnosed with cancer. You know that this diagnosis will change your life—or maybe it already has—and you are seeking guidance for the months ahead. Or perhaps, a family member or friend has been diagnosed with cancer, and you are not sure how to talk about the situation and be supportive during care. While this book is designed to guide anyone who studies health communication or who deals with cancer, we hope *Conversing with Cancer* and the guidance in this book reach, either directly or indirectly, those readers who need it most: the people living with cancer, both the patient and that person's family members and friends. When we discuss the varied roles of providers—physicians, nurses, social workers—we want the patient, too, to gain useful insight into how these individuals participate in cancer care. Understanding the entire healthcare team, from formal paid providers in the healthcare system to informal, unpaid family caregivers, helps us decide how to interact so that we get the best health care and make the best decisions.

Strong communication depends on each individual in the interaction and the history of conversations and other communicative experiences brought to the current exchange. Each person must understand the situation and each other, so we intend this book for the entire group who converses about a patient's cancer. We all need this guidance.

Getting the Most Out of This Book

Conversing with Cancer is not designed to prescribe specific action but, rather, to nourish communication skills so that the patient is more confident in decisions and actions. In other words, this book is premised on the notion that, if you give people fish, they will enjoy the meal but will grow hungry again, whereas, if you teach people how to fish, they will be able to sustain themselves over the long haul. We provide principles upon which everyone involved can rely as the cancer situation changes, day to day or over a lifetime.

Conversing with Cancer sheds light on how strong communication among providers, patients, family members, and others makes the difficult process of cancer care easier so that everyone involved can make the best decisions. This book helps the patient decide which questions to ask and how to ask them, when and where to get reliable information, how to prioritize information and tasks, and how and when to share a diagnosis with others. Since there is no set formula for deciding when to share a diagnosis with a friend or ask a physician about hospice, for example, patients should consider their own backgrounds and attitudes when deciding how to seek, share, or use information. These are communication issues to which healthcare providers and caregivers also must be sensitive, though, all too often, they are not fully aware unless they have had specialized training or read this book. Health communication scholars and students are studying these issues in depth and play an increasingly important role in improving cancer care.

As you make your way through *Conversing with Cancer*, you will see how communication about cancer can provide a path to help people continue to live their absolute best and healthiest lives through the often complex and confusing process of living with cancer. We often refer to the real-life stories that others have imparted in books, on blogs, and to us in person. These stories offer insight and suggest that there is no one formula for all cancer patients. Our goal is for all of us to live our lives in the best way possible, even as we navigate the often unfamiliar and unpredictable landscape of cancer, from prevention to detection to diagnosis and through treatment, as well as into survivorship, thriving, or end-of-life.

We have divided this book into chapters and divided chapters into sections so that readers can read straight through or can pick and choose according to their priorities. Note that each chapter begins with a poem or excerpt from a poem, the subject of which is cancer care. Poetry serves as a representation of cultural attitudes and individual viewpoints and also as a form of art that employs language in a heightened or distilled manner. The poems operate as examples of ways of conversing with and about cancer and also as linguistic patterns of intellectual and emotional responses to the continuum of cancer care. Poetry, then, becomes a creative thread woven through this scholarly book.

The next four chapters focus on the patient and health communication, especially how culture, social identity, and stage of life play a role in a person's cancer care and decision-making. Chapter 2 balances breadth and depth in an extended exploration of basic health communication principles that can be applied to individual situations and interactions. That chapter uses existing research to examine what kinds of knowledge are likely to be most helpful to providers and patients and what types of resources might provide knowledge that can be used wisely. Chapter 3 demonstrates how the patient, the caregiver, and the healthcare provider can better understand the context in which the patient is living so that stronger communication can be established and better decisions can be made. Chapter 4 shows how patients can understand themselves better, especially in terms of social identity, in order to set priorities and make better decisions. This chapter might be especially enlightening for providers who've not considered their patients as individuals in addition to biomedical situations. Chapter 5 gives special attention to adapting communication and decision-making to the patient's stage of life, whether it be in childhood, in middle age, or among the elderly.

The three chapters that follow delve into the roles of healthcare organizations, healthcare providers, and informal caregivers in the cancer care process. Chapter 6 explores how the patient can navigate the maze of the healthcare system and establish a healthcare team for the best possible care. Because of the realities of cancer, the scope of this chapter is extended to introduce hospice care as a good organizational model for coordinated health care. Chapter 7 investigates how providers communicate, how patients can encourage a partnership with providers (and vice versa), and how individuals can work together to share appropriate information and improve decision-making. Chapter 8 describes the important role of informal caregivers, who are often family members or friends untrained in cancer care but with a personal stake in positive outcomes for the patient. This chapter also extends the discussion of hospice care.

Chapter 9 and Chapter 10 focus on how we talk about cancer. They examine conversational modes as well as new technologies that support cancer care. Chapter 9 explores common ways people talk about cancer, including the common battle metaphor, and suggests how patients can develop appropriate and useful ways to talk about their cancer. Chapter 10 examines current modes of communication about cancer, with special attention to the ways computer technology and the Internet have reshaped interactions among patients, physicians, other healthcare providers, and caregivers. These chapters may be especially relevant to health communication scholars and students who study the day-to-day forms of communication in which patients engage.

The final two chapters offer new evidence-based approaches and ideas related to cancer care and, as such, are especially forward thinking. Chapter 11 breaks new ground with an extension of the Baltes and Baltes (1990) selection, optimization, and compensation model for successful aging by extending the model to consider the relationship between patient and provider and applying it to the continuum of cancer care from prevention and detection through diagnosis and treatment to survivorship and end-of-life. The final chapter—the book's epilogue—considers how others have conversed and coped with cancer and how we might extend the conversation in which this book engages.

The appendices offer additional information. Here you will find a glossary of terms, a list of books mentioned in *Conversing with Cancer*, and some online resources. Some of these extra materials will be posted on the book's website, along with bonus material not found in this book. Check www.ConversingWithCancer.com for additional resources for instructors, students, physicians, patients, caregivers, and others.

We all make choices regarding communication. A cancer diagnosis heightens certain choices, which may not be easily defined as good or bad (Sparks, 2003). As a person lives *with* cancer and communicate about it, one may face difficult choices, some of which present a double bind or affect aspects of life beyond health. The experience of cancer is often a balance between hope and despair, and our goal is to help readers feel more hopeful about their powerful role in the cancer care process. *Conversing with Cancer* can increase awareness of and ability to make necessary choices, to manage difficult turns when faced with an obstacle, and to continue on.

References

Bearman, G., Bryant, K., Leekha, S., Mayer, J., Munoz-Proce, L. S., Murthy, R., Palmore, T., Rupp, M. E., & White, J. (2014). Healthcare personnel attire in non-operating-room settings. *Infection Control and Hospital Epidemiology*, 35, 107–121.

Berger, J. (2013). *Contagious: Why things catch on*. New York, NY: Simon & Schuster.

Day, M. (2006). Doctors are told to ditch "disease spreading" neckties. *BMJ*, *332*, 442.

Jain, S. L. (2013). *Malignant: How cancer becomes us*. Oakland, CA: University of California Press.

The Joint Commission Center for Transforming Healthcare (2012). Transitions of care: The need for a more effective approach to continuing patient care. Retrieved from http://www.jointcommission.org/assets/1/18/hot_topics_transitions_of_care.pdf

Kreps, G. L., & Sparks, L. (2015). Cancer communication. In G. A. Colditz (Ed.), *The encyclopedia of cancer and society* (2nd ed., pp. 220–225). Newbury Park, CA: Sage.

Milgram, S. (1963). Behavioral study of obedience. *Journal of Abnormal and Social Psychology*, 67, 371–378.

Parrott, R. (2004). Emphasizing "communication" in health communication. *Journal of Communication*, 54, 751–757.

Sparks, L. (2003). An introduction to cancer communication and aging: Theoretical and research insights. *Health Communication*, *15*, 123–132.

Sparks, L. (2013). Health communication and caregiving research, policy, and practice. *Caregiving across the professions: A multi-disciplinary, coordinated perspective*. New York, NY: Springer.

Sparks, L. (2014). Social identity and health: An intergroup approach. In W. Donsbach (Ed.), *The international Encyclopedia of communication* (Vol. 4, pp. 1287–1290). Oxford: Wiley-Blackwell.

Sparks, L., & Nussbaum, J. F. (2008). Health literacy and cancer communication with older adults. *Patient Education and Counseling, 71*, 345–350.

Sparks, L., & Villagran, M. (2008). *La Comunicación en el Cancer: Comunicación y apoyo emocional en el laberinto del cancer*. [English translation: Communication and emotional support in the cancer maze.] Madrid, Spain: Aresta.

Sparks, L., & Villagran, M. (2010). *Patient and provider interaction: A global health communication perspective*. Cambridge, UK: Polity Press.

Sparks, L., & Villagran, M. (2014). Family caregiving. In W. Donsbach (Ed.), *The international encyclopedia of communication* (Vol. 4, pp. 488–490). Oxford: Wiley-Blackwell.

Wright, K. B., Sparks, L., & O'Hair, H. D. (2013). *Health communication in the 21st century* (2nd ed.). Oxford: Blackwell.

Zhang, J. (2010). The sound of silence: Observational learning in the UK kidney market. *Marketing Science*, *29*, 315–335.

· 2 ·

TALK, TALK

Understanding Health Communication, Health Literacy, and Cancer

> It was a warning, not cancer, not this time—
> just a little growth, a fleshy, blooming soul
> that filled my uterus, new life mimed.
> It was a warning, not cancer, not this time
> or the time before, but leaking blood and slime
> can't be ignored if certain death is not a goal.
> It was a warning, not cancer, not this time—
> just a little growth, a fleshy, blooming soul.
> —"Triolet on Beating the Odds" by Lanette Cadle

"Cancer" wasn't a word that belonged in my life: that's what I seriously thought. Though my sister Linda had lovingly badgered me over the years to go get a regular check-up, to get my first mammogram, I still felt invincible. For the first 46 years of my life, my body had served me so well. It had run marathons and won state championships. I could walk 10 or 12 miles at a stretch without protest and take all the hard yoga classes. I fed it well; I took care of it.

"But here's the truth: I do have breast cancer. I was diagnosed on March 19, 2014."

When fiction writer Patricia Grace King was diagnosed with cancer, she had not seen a doctor in nine years. Suddenly, as this excerpt from her blog reveals,

Patricia was thrust into what seemed to her like a new state of being and a new environment, one filled with healthcare professionals she had never met before, words and terminology she had never heard or said before, physically invasive tests that included needle biopsies, and numerous unexpected—and unbidden—decisions to make. Like any patient with a new cancer diagnosis, she had to acclimate to this unfamiliar, unasked-for situation as quickly as she possibly could. She had to learn how to understand what she was being told by doctors, nurses, technicians, and billing staff, and she had to learn how to talk about cancer with each of those individuals, as well as with family and friends. She had to sort through responses from colleagues and students; friends, including those who were shocked and those with their own cancer stories; and family, including her oncologist uncle who had been conversing with others' cancer for years. Patricia had to become more literate about the healthcare system and also about her disease as part of an understanding of health generally and her own health in particular. Patricia's husband had to learn new forms of communication and sort through complicated information and emotions right along with her.

A cancer *diagnosis*—the act of identifying a disease, disorder, or medical condition—often creates a situation of uncertainty, ambiguity, misunderstood information, high emotion, and anguish (Sparks, 2003, 2007, 2013). Faced with this situation, patients must make important decisions about their health care and treatment. Without strong communication and the ability to access, understand, and sort through information, the outcome of these decisions can be less positive than recent medical advances might allow. A cancer patient needs to strengthen health literacy and health communication skills to better understand and cope with the individual situation, apply information and advice appropriately, and make the best decisions possible.

In order to examine existing research in these areas of health communication and health literacy in relation to the continuum of cancer care and to provide the foundation for the chapters that follow, this chapter understandably runs longer than some others. It begins with working definitions and a theoretical framework for health communication, and then moves into definitions of types of health literacy and strategies for strengthening health literacy, particularly in relation to the continuum of cancer care.

Health Communication: A Scholarly Discipline and a Cancer Patient's Strategy

Health Communication: A Working Definition

Most people have some experience in health communication and health literacy because most of us have visited a doctor about an illness or ailment at some point across our lifespan or perhaps we have read an article or watched a television show about nutrition or exercise. While some people engage minimally with the healthcare system, perhaps because of good health or because of lack of access, others are more attentive to recommendations for routine medical care and have a relationship with a general practitioner before a serious illness, such as cancer, occurs. When Patricia started a one-year fellowship at the University of Wisconsin, she received general information about the health care provided there, specific materials that encouraged a routine check-up, and basic facts about health insurance. She was already participating in what experts call *health communication*. She did not think about these initial nudges as health communication, but whenever we engage in interactions—whenever we give or receive information—about our health or about the healthcare system, we are engaging in health communication. This receiving and giving of information about health affects us throughout our lives, and the authors of *Conversing with Cancer* have been studying how that can play a positive role in cancer care.

Health communication includes patient–provider interactions such as conversations about an individual's health history or a disease's treatment options, physical examinations and medical screenings, and even appointment reminders. Health communication can also include a billboard you see on your way to work, a brochure you receive in the mail, a casual conversation with your neighbor, the GPS directions to the Emergency Room, a television show in which a character gets cancer, a social media post from a friend or family member, as well as a host of other modes for giving and receiving information.

Sometimes, health communication seems a simple thing; it is not something most people work to improve because they do not tend to think about it as a skill. But it is an important life skill, and developing health communication skills can help whether a person is a patient, a caregiver, or a provider. In cancer care, the receiving and giving of health information is especially important because it affects real individual lives threatened by disease. Health communication about cancer often begins before diagnosis, perhaps when seeing a warning on a pack of cigarettes or in an airport jet way or when a friend is diagnosed with cancer. Even negotiating the pre-diagnosis phase can be difficult. A cancer diagnosis heightens the need for strong communication.

Often, people do not apply information about routine health care to their own health situations. In other words, even when we know to eat healthy or to have a screening mammogram, we do not consciously think: *that applies to me right now*. Sometimes, different healthcare organizations, providers, or friends present seemingly contradictory information, which can make it more difficult to know how health information applies to an individual and for that person to take the action that is best.

According to the National Cancer Institute (NCI), for instance, *mammograms*—x-ray imaging used to detect breast cancer—are less effective in detecting cancer in younger breasts and in dense breasts. In addition, younger, denser breast tissue is more easily damaged by the x-rays of a mammogram, which, especially with repeated exposure, increases the risk of developing cancer (see Fact Sheet). That is why women in their twenties rarely get mammograms; the risk of radiation exposure over the remaining lifetime outweighs the chance of detecting cancer in women who are younger. Experts tend to agree on this basic health information. In fact, the NCI recently changed its general recommendation to take into account this new information about age and breast density; it now recommends that, for most women without a family history of breast cancer, screening mammograms can begin at age 50 (see Fact Sheet). The American Cancer Society, however, still recommends mammograms starting at age 40 because mammography has been an effective screening tool and because early diagnosis plays an important role in breast cancer survival (Breast Cancer). Even though the two organizations do not disagree on the facts or research findings, each has a slightly different general recommendation for the right age to start regular screening mammograms. Both advocate screening mammograms, and both agree that a particular individual may want to begin screenings earlier or later than recommended. These organizations, therefore, encourage each woman to talk with her physician so that she can make the best decision based on her family health history, age, breast tissue density, and other factors. Healthcare organizations provide general information—or messaging—and structure, and providers apply research and experience to an individual patient.

When Patricia called to arrange her visit for general health care, she had felt an unusual solid ridge in her breast but hoped it was nothing. She mentioned it when she called to schedule a checkup but hoped that she would not need a mammogram yet. Maybe Patricia was following the NCI guidelines that led her to wait until she was fifty years old to begin annual screening mammograms, but she had not talked with a healthcare provider about whether that general recommendation applied to her situation. Patricia never had a screening mammogram. Because Patricia had already felt something unusual in her breast, her first mammogram was not routine; it was considered diagnostic because the radiologist was looking for something that already could be felt. The person who scheduled her appointment informed Patricia that her mammogram would be done at an imaging center, one of the many types of organizations in the healthcare system and one of many places on the map of that healthcare facility. In this way, Patricia entered cancer care even before her diagnosis and was already engaged in health communication that would be the foundation of her cancer care.

Health Literacy: A Working Definition

The ability to access, understand, sort through, and use information or advice about health is referred to as *health literacy*. Health communication skills and health literacy are important for everyone to develop because health communication affects every person. An individual can benefit from understanding how general recommendations, research findings, treatment options, and other health information apply to one's specific situation. Health communication includes the information and messages a person receives and gives and also the mode of interaction that transfers that information or message.

Health literacy is grounded in health communication, and both are important for the cancer patient throughout the process of living with and beyond cancer (Kreps, Neuhauser, Sparks, & Villagran, 2008; Kreps & Sparks, 2008; Sparks & Nussbaum, 2008; Wright, Sparks, & O'Hair, 2013). Communication about cancer involves deciding which questions to ask and when to ask them, where to get reliable information that can inform decisions, and how or when to share the diagnosis with others. Literacy is not only about having a lot of information, but also about knowing how to organize and evaluate that information so that you can use it in interactions and decision-making.

You almost certainly will not know all the medical and cancer lingo before you or someone close to you is diagnosed with cancer. S. Lochlann Jain (2013) recounts the information she received a week after her diagnosis: a pathology report. "Abbreviated as 'path report,' this description of the removed tissue joins other morsels of cancer lingo, such as the conversion of stomach-wrenching chemotherapy into the too-familiar 'chemo,' the more manageable 'mets' or 'hotspots' for life-threatening metastases" (p. 7). There is little chance someone like Jain would know what *hotspots* were in cancer care prior to direct experience with cancer. Literacy does not mean knowing everything about a topic. The goal of health literacy is, in part, for people to know how to learn what they need to know—learn how to acquire information and knowledge—in order to be more active and more positive in their own health care.

The ever-changing and evolving landscape of populations in the United States challenges providers and researchers to adapt existing research efforts to reflect the needs of an increasingly diverse society and to make concerted efforts toward reducing health disparities (Napoles-Springer, Santoyo-Olsson, & O'Brien, 2006; Smedley, Stith, & Nelson, 2003; Sparks & Miller-Day, 2014). The term *health disparity* suggests difference, inequality, and unfairness in the quality and access to health care among different population groups (LeCook, McGuire, & Zaslavsky, 2012) and often involves differences in direct health care, operation of healthcare systems, legal and regulatory climates, discrimination, and other factors (Institute of Medicine, 2003; LeCook et al., 2012). While much of the literature on health disparities focuses on race, ethnicity, and socioeconomic status, there are a variety of other cultural groups experiencing inequities in health care including the elderly, the LGBTQIA+ community, those with disability, as well as rural and many inner-city urban populations. As the demographic trends in the United States change, meeting the needs of diverse cultural groups becomes more challenging and vital, and adaptations to traditional communication approaches are warranted. Health literacy and competent cultural communication efforts that reflect *cultural diversity*—a variety of cultural or ethnic groups or individuals—and enhance rich cultural exchanges can dramatically reduce disparities and increase health outcomes.

Communication scholars have been working to find ways to encourage health literacy and communication that fosters emotional and medical support, nourishes interactions with healthcare professionals and friends, and helps cancer patients live their best and healthiest lives. This work is ongoing, and readers of this book can carry forward ways to improve health literacy and communication in their lives and in the larger healthcare system. This chapter sheds light on how communication among patients, providers, family members, and other sources, including the Internet, can enhance the difficult process of cancer care. That way, we can all make the best health decisions and, as such, live our lives in the best way possible as we navigate the often uncertain, complex, and confusing world of *conversing with cancer*.

Theoretical Framework

Lifespan Relational Communication Health Theory

You are involved in many, many interactions every day that build over time to create who you are and how you interact and connect with your relationships across your lifespan. When you kiss your spouse or wake your child, that is an interaction that communicates. When you listen to classical music on the radio as you brew your coffee in the morning, that is also a form of nonverbal communication. When it comes down to it, even the "brew" button on your coffee maker and your knowledge of what to do with it creates a communication interaction. Conversations, text messages, street signs, recipes, and a host of other information exchanges we take for granted as daily life are all interactions that communicate information.

The underlying framework for this book and our approach to communication and literacy about cancer is a kind of social health theory we call *lifespan relational communication health theory*. This approach builds upon and hones prior ideas of social health theory as described by Lisa Sparks and colleagues (e.g., Sparks & Villagran, 2008, 2009, 2010). The central premise of lifespan relational communication health theory is that a person's conversations and history of interactions over long-term relationships and over time create, maintain, and/or destroy relationships in positive and negative ways that, across the life span, ultimately can affect our health (Bevan & Sparks, 2011, 2013; Sparks & Villagran, 2008, 2009, 2010). These interactions may include early conversations with one's mother about eating all the vegetables on the dinner plate or instructions received in elementary school about brushing one's teeth. When someone sees a general practitioner or a medical specialist, those interactions—conversations, examinations, tests, test results, and so on—shape and reshape the patient's attitudes, behaviors, and health.

So, when this book uses the framework of lifespan relational communication health theory to understand and talk about cancer, it builds on the idea that communication exchanges over time have an impact on relationships and that relationships have an impact on communication exchanges. After all, it is through our relationships with others that we most often seek health information, obtain guidance about health, and make decisions about how to improve health and treat illness (Sparks, 2013; Sparks & Villagran, 2010). Research indicates, for instance, that health literacy can be combined with family interactions to promote cancer screenings. An examination of the associations among socio-demographic factors, family communication, and cancer literacy in a diverse population suggests that family-centered networks may be a useful and perhaps powerful means for sharing health cancer literacy information, may inform cancer care decision-making, and may contribute to decreasing breast and cervical cancer mortality (Zambrana et al., 2015).

Mary Lee Leahy, the mother of one of this book's authors, is a good example of how interactions over a lifetime affected attitudes toward health and health care. She had many surgeries as a child but was too young to understand all that was going on, so even as an adult, her blood pressure would rise as soon as she entered a doctor's office. By the end of the visit, after conversations with the nurse and the physician and when she knew she would be leaving soon, Mary Lee's blood pressure would return to normal. During doctor visits, she had her blood pressure measured after she had interacted with the healthcare providers, when she felt more at ease. Mary Lee's individual history of interactions with the healthcare system profoundly affected every interaction with healthcare professionals and healthcare facilities all her life, including during her cancer care. Because she was aware of her tendency to be extremely uncomfortable in healthcare environments, she consciously focused on developing clear, honest ways of talking with her new healthcare providers and on applying communication skills she used in other areas of her life to her cancer care.

That is just one example of how communication impacts our health over time. Each day, we make conscious and unconsciousness choices about the people with whom we interact. All these interactions are communication acts that affect our attitudes and behaviors. Some interactions will be positive and some will be negative. The daily goal, based on our life-span approach, is to consciously choose to engage in more positive interactions than negative interactions, thereby creating more positive and healthy relationships in our lives. With more positive relationships, attitudes, and behaviors, we are better equipped to make good health decisions, make the best decisions when faced with cancer, and successfully age (Sparks & Nussbaum, 2008).

Offsetting Negative Interactions and Outlooks

At the same time, we must consciously let go of as many negative interactions as possible throughout all areas of our lives. For instance, if a person has a negative interaction during the day, that individual should try to engage with at least an equal number of positive, healthy interactions before the end of the day (Sparks & Villagran, 2008, 2009, 2010). Consciously do this each and every day, and you will slowly lessen or rid yourself of the relationships that are contributing negatively to your life and, by extension, your health. Research indicates that increasing positive interactions and decreasing negative interactions will likely result in living the healthiest, best possible life (Bevan & Sparks, 2011, 2013). When someone is living with cancer—whether you are living as a patient, a caregiver, or a provider—this approach to communication can play an important role in the cancer care process.

Continuing research is needed to more fully understand the function of *life-span interaction health theory* in terms of how exactly our health is affected in positive and negative ways as a result of our interactions with our environment over time. That said, because cancer treatment can sometimes seem like one negative experience after another, we are suggesting that patients begin to consciously offset as many of those as possible with more positive interactions and relationships to achieve a more satisfactory and, arguably, a healthier way of life as they negotiate cancer care. As Sparks and Villagran (2010) argue, we suggest that it is important pay attention to the positive interactions in daily life and especially across a lifespan and to consciously spend more time nurturing those relationships that are contributing to your life in positive and healthy ways.

That said, offsetting negative experiences should not suggest that a person should deny the seriousness of a situation. Some interactions, such as the initial cancer diagnosis, are inherently negative. To dismiss that reality can inadvertently make a patient feel trivialized or criticized. As Barbara Ehrenreich (2010) notes in *Bright-Sided: How the Relentless Promotion of Positive Thinking Has Undermined America*, "It could be argued that positive thinking can't hurt, that it might even be a blessing to the sorely afflicted" (p. 40). That said, she goes on to discuss possible harms of promoting positive thinking without context and understanding of individual circumstances:

> First, it requires the denial of understandable feelings of anger and fear, all of which must be buried under a cosmetic layer of cheer. This is a great convenience

> for health workers and even friends of the afflicted, who might prefer fake cheer to complaining, but it is not so easy on the afflicted. [...]
>
> Besides, it takes effort to maintain the upbeat demeanor expected by others [...].

These considerations lead us to suggest offsetting negative interactions rather than merely avoiding the unwelcome reality of cancer or stifling genuine complaints or symptoms of pain and fatigue. Avoidance and faking it are rarely good for communication and can undermine health care. Because negative experiences cannot be completely avoided in life—and are part of life with cancer—welcoming and seeking positive experiences is often part of healthful living.

Building Positive Interactions and Outlooks

Without discounting the seriousness of negative interactions, patients may find positive aspects of the experience or may shift their outlook to try to offset the negative aspects. Patricia King was shocked and disbelieving when she first heard from a physician that she had breast cancer. But she had access to a great healthcare facility that provided her with clear next steps. And phone conversations with her oncologist uncle reassured her and even convinced her to write about and share this experience that, at face value, seemed utterly awful.

Likewise, Amanda Niehaus was diagnosed with breast cancer at the age of 31, just after celebrating her first Mother's Day as a mother herself. She holds a post-doctoral fellowship at the University of Queensland in Australia, where she studies, on the metabolic and cellular levels, how marsupials age and die. As a response to her own cancer diagnosis, treatment, and survival, she started writing the blog *Easy Peasy Organic* because she wanted to communicate about healthful and maintainable ways to eat and live. There, she wrote:

> breast cancer *has* opened doors, and defined me, in unexpected ways. I'm not going to say that it was the greatest thing ever to happen to me {because it wasn't—it was shit}, or that it was worth it for all I learned {because I was blissfully happy being immortal}. But I have learned from cancer, I have gained from it.

Six years after her diagnosis, Amanda writes about health, happiness, eating well, and what science means. No one wants cancer, but Amanda's experience with cancer led her to become involved in health advocacy, a powerful form of health communication that connects information, behavior, and lifestyle to promote positive health outcomes.

Many people may not, of course, have spent much time thinking about the connection between communication, relationships, health, and cancer. In order to become a well-educated consumer of health information as a cancer patient, an individual must become more literate about health and especially about cancer and also gain a deeper understanding of how communicative interactions and relationships can play a crucial role in health in a variety of ways. Having cancer makes health communication and literacy all the more important to a person's well-being over time, but health communication and literacy is important for anyone who strives to live the best life.

The Importance of Health Literacy in Health Communication

Health literacy, as we have mentioned, is the level of mastery that individuals have in finding, judging, and understanding health information and health-care services so that they can make the best decisions about their health (Kreps et al., 2008; O'Hair, Kreps, & Sparks, 2007). While most people interact with health information and make decisions that affect their health throughout their entire lives, according to the U.S. Department of Health and Human Services ("Quick Guide to Health Literacy," which cites a study by Kirsh et al. [1993]), few are very capable in this area of life:

> Only 12 percent of adults have *proficient* health literacy, according to the National Assessment of Adult Literacy. In other words, nearly 9 out of 10 adults may lack the skills needed to manage their health and prevent disease. Fourteen percent of adults (30 million people) have *below basic* health literacy. These adults were more likely to report their health as poor (42 percent) and are more likely to lack health insurance (28 percent) than adults with *proficient* health literacy. Low literacy has been linked to poor health outcomes such as higher rates of hospitalization and less frequent use of preventive services. (italics ours)

Drawing from a 2003 survey, *The Health Literacy of America's Adults* (2006) also points out that Hispanic adults and older adults have lower than average health literacy, pointing to ways identity intersects with health care. Health literacy—clear communication and understanding of information—can greatly influence patient safety and health outcomes. For a cancer patient, becoming more informed and managing information and interaction can matter both day to day and over the long term.

The Joint Commission Center for Transforming Healthcare, in the article "Transitions of Care: The Need for a More Effective Approach to Continuing Patient Care," points to a study that "estimated that 80 percent of serious medical errors involve miscommunication during the hand-off between medical providers" (see also Sparks & Nussbaum, 2008). Miscommunication and lack of interaction have serious consequences. That is a powerful call for improved communication among healthcare providers, of course, and also a call for patients to become more literate and skilled in health communication so that they can participate actively in decision-making and coordination of care.

The root causes of this miscommunication include communication breakdown between providers and between provider and patient, patient education issues or lack of health literacy, and accountability issues that occur especially when numerous healthcare providers are involved in a single patient's care, as is the case with cancer patients (Sparks, 2011; Sparks & Villagran, 2008, 2009, 2010; Wright et al., 2013). For someone with cancer, therefore, improving the ability to communicate about health, increasing health literacy through education and by seeking out information, and looking for signs of coordination problems among the healthcare providers can lead to fewer serious problems as patients make decisions and move through treatment. In fact, in Chapters 6 through 8, we discuss in more detail the roles of healthcare organizations, healthcare providers, and caregivers and how a patient can coordinate and communicate with everyone involved in one's cancer care.

Health literacy is key to underpinning all these interactions. It is one major factor that determines how an individual navigates the healthcare system, how a person obtains health information, and how well that person understands preventative practices and choices. Increasing health literacy through strong communication can help a person change behaviors to lower the risk of getting cancer, negotiate the healthcare system more deftly, make important decisions after a cancer diagnosis, and avoid problems as one continues to deal with cancer over weeks, months, and years of health care.

Many physicians continue to take a routine and biomedical approach to patients, rather than using an approach tailored to each individual case and each patient's needs. Research suggests, however, that, when physicians are perceived as more patient-centered and as better communicators, their patients are more satisfied and more likely to comply with provider guidance

(Street, Gordon, & Haidet, 2007). That same research by Street et al. (2007) also indicates that physicians who are attentive to a patient's level of health literacy tend to communicate better with patients as individual people.

There exist many ways for individuals and communities to increase health literacy. Health literacy can be considered as encompassing the following four aspects (Sparks & Villagran, 2010; Sparks, O'Hair, & Kreps, 2008): cultural and conceptual knowledge, oral literacy, print literacy, and numeracy. Both patients and providers engage in all four aspects or modes of health literacy.

Cultural and Conceptual Knowledge

Cultural and conceptual knowledge refers to the big picture understanding and to the knowledge we have about health care that we seem to acquire without effort along the way or sometimes take for granted. A person may pick up information about how hospitals work or that physicians specialize in different kinds of medicine, for instance, from watching news media or film or television entertainment (e.g., *August: Osage County*, *W;t*, *Brian's Song*, *Breaking Bad*, *Chicago Hope*, *ER*, *Philadelphia*, *Homeland*, *Nurse Jackie*, *The Big C*, *House*, *Grey's Anatomy*, *Terms of Endearment*, *50/50*, *The Bucket List*, *The Bold and the Beautiful*, *Dying Young*, *My Life*, *Stepmom*). You may know that exercise is good for your health without remembering where you learned that; you may exercise because you spend time with other people who tend to value exercise for recreation and social interaction as well as for its health benefits, not because you are consciously thinking about improving your own health and lowering your risk of disease.

Communities—neighborhoods, schools, cities, television viewing audiences—can foster this sort of broad knowledge about health. A city may encourage exercise by offering relatively easy access to attractive open spaces with free admission to biking, hiking, and running trails. Further, every geographical community can and should provide places where people can easily get checkups for their own health needs and can encourage *cancer prevention*, or the use of active behaviors to reduce cancer risk. A community might teach new parents about the importance of putting sunscreen on their toddlers every day, thereby establishing lifelong healthy habits. In 2000, when television anchor Katie Couric, whose husband had died of colon cancer, underwent her own colonoscopy as part of the *Today Show*, general awareness of the disease increased at least temporarily, and, according to a report in *Archives of Internal*

Medicine by Cram et al. (2003), more people sought the screening procedure for colorectal cancer.

Cultural and conceptual knowledge is shared knowledge and often knowledge that we take for granted or that seems intuitive or common sense. Sharing reliable health information so that it becomes cultural or conceptual knowledge is the responsibility of the larger community as well as individuals within it.

Oral Literacy

Oral literacy refers to the information we have heard or discussed, information we share through listening or speaking, everywhere and all the time. Some of us learned about the importance of eating fruits and vegetables from a teacher or parent. You may have asked about a bump or rash that appeared on your skin or talked with friends about a certain kind of pain that concerned you. Both the ability to ask questions verbally and understand what healthcare professionals say in response is part of oral literacy. Understanding vocabulary and medical terminology, picking up on inflection and body language, and addressing confusion all play a role in increasing oral health literacy and improving communication.

Print Literacy

Print literacy involves what we write and what we read. Warnings on cigarette labels, shower cards demonstrating a breast self-exam, a brochure on colorectal cancer, and an explanation of benefits from an insurance company are all forms of print information geared to improve health literacy. A list of symptoms you write down and even a personal journal fit into the concept of health literacy as well. When Mary Lee Leahy (the author's mother) was scheduled for a biopsy of her pancreas, she went online to search for and read information about pancreatic cancer even before the diagnosis had been confirmed. She was using her print—or textual—literacy to gather and organize information.

Findings from a 2003 health literacy survey (*The Health Literacy of America's Adults*, 2006) of people 16 years of age and older reveal that many adults, unlike Mary Lee, have limited print literacy, even with everyday materials such as magazines, and are less likely to use print materials with accuracy and consistency. Understanding the language and terminology used is crucial for understanding information. Internet information or brochures may introduce confusion when unfamiliar words are used and immediate clarification is not typically available. In addition, though healthcare providers may assume that printed information in English serves most patients well, a patient or caregiver who grew up in Mexico may speak English well but find information printed in Spanish much easier to understand and remember. Cancer patients should ask their healthcare providers for clarification about any print information that is confusing. In fact, follow-up conversations can be helpful because patients may not realize they have misinterpreted a statement. Extended and ongoing communication can allow everyone involved in communicative interactions to see and address gaps in knowledge.

This chapter focuses on health literacy. How can you judge whether you are *cancer literate*? Here are a few questions to consider as one navigates the complex and often confusing information about cancer.

- How would you describe your own health literacy right now? What obstacles do you have to becoming more literate? What motivates you to become more informed about health issues or your own health?
- Are there medical terms you have read or heard that you are not sure you understand? Is it easy or difficult for you to put relevant medical information into your own words and apply it to a specific situation?
- How significant do you think patient–provider communication is in preventing cancer, detecting cancer, diagnosing cancer, treating cancer, surviving cancer, and end-of-life issues?
- How do you think patient–provider communication should be evaluated? What methods and measures would use to assess whether patient–provider communication is strong or weak?
- What behaviors or statements do you look for to recognize confusion in others? If confusion occurs in conversation or online exchange, what do you usually do? What would you do if you were in the other person's shoes?
- Describe the provider's role in supporting communication between patient and caregiver. What is the provider's responsibility in an interaction about cancer care? What is the patient's responsibility?

Numeracy

Numeracy may be the most intimidating area of literacy for many cancer patients because many of us are not as accustomed in our daily lives to think in or interpret numbers. Some patients will have to sort through information about insurance co-payments, deductibles, and out-of-pocket expenses or negotiate the intricacies of Medicare, Medicaid, or socialized healthcare payment systems. Many patients will seek out statistics about cancer risk and long-term survival. Knowledge about this sort of numeric data, including statistics, is *numeracy* (Weber, Sparks, & LaBelle, 2015).

Most lung cancer results from smoking, and 80% of lung cancer deaths are attributed to smoking. "But risk factors don't tell us everything," as the American Cancer Society (2016) says about lung cancer. "Having a risk factor, or even several risk factors, does not mean that you will get the disease. And some people who get the disease may not have had any known risk factors." This language is from a report called "What Are the Risk Factors for Getting Small Cell Lung Cancer?" Note, though, that the American Cancer Society uses this language in many informational materials about different types of cancer in an attempt to help patients understand that, regardless of the type of cancer, statistics are about groups not about individuals.

That number—80% of lung cancer deaths result from smoking—is powerful because we understand it as a large percentage. But it does not tell us anything about how many individual smokers develop lung cancer, how long those who get cancer smoked, nor anything about survival rates. Again, statistics are about groups, not about individuals. Statistics do not predict exactly what will happen to *you* because statistics are typically reporting the mean (average) or median (midpoint, with 50% of instances above and below), and your situation may be what is referred to as a statistical outlier and not around the mean or median that the study results are describing.

It is a good idea for a patient to talk with healthcare professionals to understand what the numbers—level of risk, statistics about treatment effectiveness, dosages for medicine, insurance co-pays and deductibles, and so on—mean specifically for that patient's treatment.

Treatment choices are often made in an environment of uncertainty, ambiguity, misunderstood information, high emotion, and anguish. As a result, the outcome of these choices can be less favorable than recent medical advances could allow. Communication must keep up with medical advances. It is also very important to increase levels of health literacy—cultural and conceptual knowledge, oral literacy, print literacy, and numeracy—in order to strengthen health communication. Only then can each and every cancer patient make the best decisions possible even though the circumstances may be very stressful.

Building Health Literacy: Finding and Evaluating Sources of Information

Let's say you have a family member who has just been diagnosed with colon cancer. Let's say also that you are a well-educated and curious person, so you are able to gather various kinds of health information about cancer by talking with doctors and other healthcare providers, by contacting friends who know someone with colon cancer, and through online searches. Those are all examples of ways to find health information. You spend time learning new terms and definitions, ways to talk about the diagnosis, possible treatment options, and directions for specific treatment or care tasks. You definitely are becoming more literate about your family member's cancer care situation with each passing day.

You may find lots of general information, but you may not know which of it applies to a loved one's situation. You process as much information as possible. Sometimes you come across conflicting information from different providers, friends' anecdotes, and various websites. Sometimes, you search for hours or even over days without finding exactly what you are looking for. And some of the information is difficult to understand because it uses technical language not familiar to you. Despite your improving health literacy, the information, at times, remains overwhelming and confusing in terms of how it applies to your family member and what exactly is the best choice about what should be done. You need to sort through that information so that it makes sense for you.

Not every source, of course, is a credible and reliable source of health information. Gathering information is the first step, but analyzing the information to consider credibility and inconsistencies is the next step. Consider who wrote the information—and why. Do not take every piece of information at face value. Then, consider the individual situation and whether the information applies—and how. The following two questions should guide you:

1) Is the information reliable?
2) Is the information applicable to this person and this situation?

You may have heard advice to put butter on a burn, but that advice is not very reliable; butter applied immediately to a burn can cause additional tissue damage by trapping the heat. You may have heard that you should not text while you drive, and that is reliable information based on research, but many people do not think it applies to them and fail to take simple steps to safeguard their own health and the health of others. You may have heard that vigorous exercise is good for you, and for many people it can be, but those who have osteoporosis and a history of bone fractures should avoid certain types of high-impact exercise. You may have heard *chemotherapy*—cancer-fighting chemical drugs—causes vomiting, and that is true of some chemotherapy drugs; not all of them cause nausea, however, and those for which that side effect is listed do not cause vomiting in all patients. All these examples demonstrate how both reliability and applicability of information are important in health care.

These questions—reliability and applicability—are separate tests of information and equally important as one gathers, sorts, and uses advice and information. Only then can someone use the information to make the best decisions.

For instance, you may find reliable statistics about cancer risk or survival. When Mary Lee looked online at the survival rates immediately after her pancreatic cancer diagnosis, it was easy to lose all hope. She knew information from a federal agency was reliable and based on analysis of large populations. But while one person with pancreatic cancer may have a tumor that cannot be removed, another may be a good candidate for the Whipple surgery that improves the chance for longer-term survival. In addition, an individual patient may have characteristics that may result in a stronger health outcome: age, overall physical health status, genetic predispositions, tolerance for certain medications and treatments, and so on. Though Mary Lee was already in her early seventies when diagnosed, she was in very good general health and taking few medications. Importantly, her cancer had not *metastasized*, or spread to other areas of the body, though she did not know this information about her specific situation when she first started gathering general information online. Health information needs to be considered in relation to the individual cancer patient's situation (see Mukamel, Wenzel, Ladd, Osann, Havrilesky, Sparks, et al. 2017; Mukamel, Wenzel, Ladd, Osann, Havrilesky, Wright, et al. 2017).

How can people increase the likelihood that they will be able to find what they need, understand information they acquire, and accomplish attainable goals in cancer care? For patients to reach a high level of cancer literacy, healthcare providers and healthcare systems must work with patients to create shared meaning—shared language, understanding, and priorities—that is tailored to each cancer patient. Cancer literacy is more than being able to obtain and process information and services. Literacy also prepares you for decision-making and action.

In order to encourage shared meaning, providers should offer messages in multiple mediums for the message receiver—patient, family, or caregiver. For instance, when a physician must break bad news to the patient verbally, that doctor also might provide a large-font written version or a visual-picture version of the discussion for the patient and the *caregiver*—usually the paid or familial person with significant responsibility for caring for or helping the patient—to take home. Research, in fact, supports the notion that a patient will understand health information better and be more likely to recall that information if it is presented in pictures (Kessels, 2003). Mary Lee's surgeon explained the position of a tumor on the pancreas by shaping his hand into an elongated fist to represent the pancreas and pointing to the place where the tumor was with his other hand. She could visualize what was happening inside her body. A surgeon may show the patient and the family where a tumor is located on a visual diagram of a human body and then also touch the patient's body to show where the cancer is located.

Technology, which we discuss in depth in Chapter 10, can also help patients and caregivers understand information. In her book *Everybody's Got Something*, Robin Roberts (2014) describes an interaction with her doctor in which he recognized that she did not fully understand the seriousness of her health situation. She writes:

> There was a graph showing one year and two years with a dot in the middle. He turned the computer screen so Amber [Roberts's partner and caregiver] and I could see the dot.
>
> I asked, "What's that?"
>
> At first, I thought I had one or two years to do something about what I was facing.
>
> He said, "That's your life expectancy if you don't do anything." (p. 33)

The reality was harsh, but the way her physician showed Roberts (2014) the facts and the way she asked for explanation allowed her to adjust quickly into what she calls "warrior mode" (p. 33). In Chapter 9, we talk more about the warrior and other metaphors for talking about cancer.

Varied ways of conversing about cancer give the patient and caretakers time to absorb the information and also reveal gaps in understanding that the physician can address. Communication works best when all people involved in the interaction increase their understanding of each other's literacy levels as well as of the medical information itself.

Increasing Health Literacy for Effective Communication

Patients should ask questions, and providers should take time for and encourage questions. If a physician hands a patient a brochure, we encourage that patient to ask, *Can you show me the most important information in this material?* That encourages further provider–patient interaction about that health information, creates time for specific questions to come to mind, and gives the patient and the provider a chance to tease out any hidden confusion. Patients may also want to get in the habit of asking a future-directed question toward the end of each visit, even if it as simple as: *Based on what you've told me today, what should I do next?* Or, *Is there anything else I should do before my next appointment, test, or treatment?* These future-directed questions can give a patient a clearer plan for action. Future-directed statements and questions also reinforce hope and a positive attitude by overtly reminding the provider and the patient that the person will be back.

Another way to increase literacy is for the patient to bring a spouse or another family member to appointments. This informal patient navigator should be someone the patient trusts who can be there to help the patient find a path through the information, conversations, and options. Such a person might help form a list of questions before the visit, remind the patient of questions or concerns during the visit, listen to the provider's answers, and talk with the patient about the information after the visit. Cancer patients often have numerous procedures that must be undergone as well as multiple medications to take. A navigator can help keep track of those details and also identify additional questions to ask the provider so the patient can know exactly what to do next. The navigator should always be ready to ask a simple but specific question such as: *Could you show me how to do that?*

Ideally, a cancer patient should leave the provider's office able to explain the diagnosis, treatment protocol, and/or set of issues in one's own words and also know where to go for additional information. A cancer patient should also leave the provider's office knowing how best to contact someone at the office with any additional questions. Think, for instance, how important it is in college for a student to know where and how to get clarification or additional information when working on a major assignment, perhaps from the instructor via email, on the syllabus or assignment guideline handout, or at the library. The same educational need applies to cancer care. A patient can talk in more detail later to clarify recommendations and get further information in the modes that fit the physician's schedule and the patient's needs.

Health literacy skills are not only important for people affected by cancer in general, but perhaps even more so as they are exposed to complex treatment and follow-up care information. Research indicates that radiation oncologists' understandings and awareness of health literacy among patients with a reasonable command of English can have a large impact on patient health outcomes. Within the oncology context, radiation specialists have acknowledged the importance of health literacy and have incorporated several techniques—analogies, drawings, qualitative adjectives (instead of percentages), etc.—so that they can adjust their interpersonal communication to meet the needs of groups with varying levels of literacy (Smith, Petrak, Dhillon, Taylor, & Milross, 2014). We discuss this sort of cultural competence and related issues further in Chapter 3.

Health communication can empower patients and give patients choices in modes of information gathering, understanding, and processing. Providers and caregivers, too, must work to improve communication and have clear, honest interactions. Only then can each cancer patient make the best decisions possible and lead the best life. Health literacy and health communication work reciprocally, each strengthening the other over a lifespan of interactions.

Exercise & Discussion

There is so much information out there that it is incredibly overwhelming for people who have just been diagnosed with cancer to evaluate all the information online, on television, in books, and in magazines and newspapers. Instead of merely stating a diagnosis, doctors should also give recommendations for information resources. What resources would you recommend? Note that you may need to do some research in order to recommend useful resources.

- Which websites and online forums might a patient visit for reliable information about how health care works and about cancer in particular?
- What physical places might a patient or caregiver visit to seek or find helpful information?

- What three books or movies might guide a patient in thinking about one's own diagnosis and treatment? What do you think those resources convey to readers or viewers who have cancer?
- What three articles might provide guidance in a patient's search for information about a cancer diagnosis?
- How might a physician educate patients with low health literacy or someone who has not seen a physician in ten years about different treatment options, such as radiation and chemotherapy? How would a physician change the approach to meet the needs of a moderately literate patient or someone who gets regular checkups? How might one physician inform another physician-turned-patient of a cancer diagnosis?
- Consider a difficult decision in your own life. What helped you make that decision?

References

American Cancer Society. (2016). What are the risk factors for getting small cell lung cancer? Retrieved from http://www.cancer.org/cancer/lungcancer-smallcell/detailedguide/small-cell-lung-cancer-risk-factors

Bevan, J., & Sparks, L. (2011). Communication in the context of long-distance family caregiving: An integrated review and practical applications. *Patient Education and Counseling*, *85*, 26–30.

Bevan, J., & Sparks, L. (2013). The relationship between accurate and benevolently biased serial argument perceptions and individual negative health perceptions. *Communication Research*, *41*, 257–281.

Cram, P., Frederick, A. M., Inadomi, J., Cowen, M. E., Carpenter, D., & Vijan, S. (2003). The impact of a celebrity promotional campaign on the use of colon cancer screening. *Archives of Internal Medicine*, *163*(13), 1601–1605.

Ehrenreich, B. (2010). *Bright-sided: How positive thinking is undermining America*. New York, NY: Picador.

Institute of Medicine. (2003). *Unequal treatment: Confronting racial and ethnic disparities in healthcare*. Washington, DC: National Academies Press.

Jain, S. L. (2013). *Malignant: How cancer becomes us*. Oakland, CA: University of California Press.

Joint Commission Center for Transforming Healthcare (2016). Transitions of care: The need for a more effective approach to continuing patient care. Retrieved from http://www.jointcommission.org/assets/1/18/hot_topics_transitions_of_care.pdf

Kessels, R. P. C. (2003). Patients' memory for medical information. *Journal of the Royal Society for Medicine* 96, 219–222.

Kirsch I. S., Jungeblut A., Jenkins L., & Kolstad A. (1993). *Adult Literacy in America: A First Look at the Results of the National Adult Literacy Survey (NALS)*. Washington, DC: National Center for Education Statistics, U.S. Department of Education.

Kreps, G. L., Neuhauser, L., Sparks, L., & Villagran, M. M. (2008). The power of community-based health communication interventions to promote cancer prevention and control for at-risk populations. *Patient Education and Counseling, 71*, 315–318.

Kreps, G. L., & Sparks, L. (2008). Meeting the health literacy needs of vulnerable populations. *Patient Education and Counseling, 71*, 328–332.

LeCook, B., McGuire, T. G., & Zaslavsky, A. M. (2012). Measuring racial/ethnic disparities in health care: Methods and practical issues. *Health Services Research, 47*, 1232–1254.

Mukamel, D. B., Wenzel, L., Ladd, H., Osann, K., Havrilesky, L., Sparks, L., Lipscomb, J., Wright A. A., Walker, J., Alvarez, R., Van Le, L., Disilvestro, K., Bristow, R., Morgan, R., Rimmel, B., Ladd, H., Hsieh, S., Wahi, A., & Cohn, D. (2017). Patients' preferences over treatment side-effects reflect a latent "optimism" characteristic. *Contemporary Clinical Trials*.

Mukamel, D. B., Wenzel, L., Ladd, H., Osann, K., Havrilesky, L. J., Wright, A. A., Walker, J., Alvarez, R., Van Le, L., Robison, K., Wakabayashi, M., Ferguson, S., Ehrisman, J., Sparks, L., Wahi, A., Hsieh, S., Lipscomb, J., & Cohn, D. E. (2017). The relationship between ovarian cancer patients' treatment side-effects preferences and "optimism" *Journal of Clinical Oncology*.

Napoles-Springer, A. M., Santoyo-Olsson, J., & O'Brien, H. (2006). Using cognitive interviews to develop surveys in diverse populations. *Medical Care, 44*, S21–S30.

National Center for Educational Statistics. (2006). The health literacy of America's adults: Results from the 2003 National Assessment of Health Literacy. Retrieved from http://nces.ed.gov/pubs2006/2006483.pdf

O'Hair, H. D., Kreps, G. L., & Sparks, L. (Eds.). (2007). *Handbook of communication and cancer care*. Cresskill, NJ: Hampton Press.

"Quick Guide to Health Literacy." U.S. Department of Health and Human Services. Retrieved from https://health.gov/communication/literacy/quickguide/factsbasic.htm

Roberts, R. (2014). *Everybody's got something*. New York, NY: Grand Central.

Smedley, B. D., Stith, A. Y., & Nelson, A. R. (Eds.). (2003). *Unequal treatment: Confronting racial and ethnic disparities in healthcare*. Washington, DC: National Academy Press.

Smith, S., Petrak, L., Dhillon, H., Taylor, J., & Milross, C. (2014). Are radiation oncologists aware of health literacy among people with cancer treated with radiotherapy? *European Journal of Cancer Care, 23*, 111–120. doi:10.1111/ecc.12111

Sparks, L. (2003). An introduction to cancer communication and aging: Theoretical and research insights. *Health Communication, 15*, 123–132.

Sparks, L. (Ed.). (2003). Cancer communication and aging [Editor of Special Issue]. *Health Communication, 15*.

Sparks, L. (2007). Cancer care and the aging patient: Complexities of age-related communication barriers. In H. D. O'Hair, G. L. Kreps, & L. Sparks (Eds.), *Handbook of communication and cancer care* (pp. 233–249). Cresskill, NJ: Hampton Press.

Sparks, L. (2011). Health risk messages and decision-making. TEDx OrangeCoast. Renee and Henry Segerstrom Concert Hall, Costa Mesa, CA. Age-related trends in utilization of the internet and electronic communication devices for coordination of cancer care in elderly patients. Retrieved from http://www.youtube.com/watch? v=d4JNyyuonko

Sparks, L. (2013). Health communication and caregiving research, policy, and practice. In R. C. Talley & S. S. Travis (Eds.), *Caregiving across the professions: A multi-disciplinary, coordinated perspective* (pp. 131–175). New York, NY: Springer.

Sparks, L., & Miller-Day, M. (2014). Methodological approaches to eliminating health disparities. In B. Whaley (Ed.), *Research methods in health communication: Principles and application* (pp. 318–336). New York, NY: Taylor and Francis.

Sparks, L., & Nussbaum, J. F. (2008). Health literacy and cancer communication with older adults. *Patient Education and Counseling, 71*, 345–350.

Sparks, L., O'Hair, H. D., & Kreps, G. L. (Eds.). (2008). *Cancer, communication and aging*. Cresskill, NJ: Hampton Press.

Sparks, L., & Villagran, M. (2008). *La Comunicación en el Cancer: Comunicación y apoyo emocional en el laberinto del cancer*. [English translation: Communication and emotional support in the cancer maze.] Madrid, Spain: Aresta.

Sparks, L., & Villagran, M. (2009). *Talking cancer*. Retrieved from www.editorialaresta.com

Sparks, L., & Villagran, M. (2010). *Patient and provider interaction: A global health communication perspective*. Cambridge: Polity Press.

Street, R. L., Jr., Gordon, H., & Haidet, P. (2007). Physicians' communication and perceptions of patients: Is it how they look, how they talk, or is it just the doctor? *Social Science and Medicine, 65*, 586–598.

Weber, K. A., Sparks, L., & LaBelle, S. (2015). The development and testing of a health specific subjective numeracy measure. Paper presented at Health Communication Division of the National Communication Association, Las Vegas, NV.

Wright, K. B., Sparks, L., & O'Hair, H. D. (2013). *Health communication in the 21st century* (2nd ed.). Oxford: Blackwell.

Zambrana, R. E., Meghea, C., Talley, C., Hammad, A., Lockett, M., & Williams, K. P. (2015). Association between family communication and health literacy among underserved racial/ethnic women. *Journal of Health Care for the Poor and Underserved, 26*(2), 391–405. doi:10.1353/hpu.2015.0034

· 3 ·

THE BIG C

Culture and Cancer Care

II. *that this too too sullied flesh*

Skin-deep and rank,
righteousness flees these organs
ripe with mortality's regret.
Wishes are hollow bones.
Even a Faustian switch
cannot remix the obvious.

III. *would melt, thaw*

Soon disease dissolves all self,
liquidates the I.
Listen for the drip of solitude
and relent. The dark waters
of doubt ebb and flow too quickly
downstream.

—from "Cancer Diagnosis"
by Marjorie Maddox

II. *que esta carne tan tan manchada*

A flor de piel y absoluta,
la rectitud huye de estos órganos
maduros con el lamento de la mortalidad.
Huesos huecos son los deseos.
Ni siquiera un trato como el de Fausto
puede remodelar lo obvio.

III. *se derrita, se deshiele*

Pronto la enfermedad lo disuelve
todo, liquida el yo.
Presta atención al goteo de la soledad
y tranquilízate. Las aguas oscuras
de la duda retroceden y fluyen de prisa
corriente abajo.

—Traducción de Rei Berroa

When Mary Lee was diagnosed with breast cancer in her early sixties, she contacted the oncologist who had treated her husband when he had cancer. Because she had many childhood experiences with surgery for club foot, Mary Lee didn't like going to the doctor. She was relieved that she could see an oncologist she already knew and trusted. In the years of follow-up appointments to check for recurrence and monitor a blood condition, her appointments were scheduled as the last of the day so that she and her oncologist could talk about local and state politics and the challenges of running a small business.

When she was diagnosed with pancreatic cancer a decade later, however, Mary Lee sought out and traveled away from home to see new physicians with more experience treating that type of cancer. Pancreatic cancer is rarer than breast cancer and has a much lower survival rate so she wanted physicians with specialized expertise. Mary Lee's relationship with her new oncologist became more open after they discovered that they were both Cubs fans and could talk about the few wins and many losses of their baseball team as well as about cancer.

Mary Lee was a practicing attorney when she was diagnosed with pancreatic cancer. For decades, she had considered herself part of a community of professionals like lawyers and physicians. She and her first oncologist, the one who treated her for breast cancer, were roughly the same age, but her second was younger, perhaps not yet as old as her own daughters. Mary Lee's first oncologist was of Italian descent, and they had talked about what it meant for him to grow up Italian-American and her to grow up Irish-American because they assumed similarities existed, whereas her second oncologist was of Pakistani heritage. In part because of these differences between Mary Lee and her new oncologist and in part because the prognosis was dire, they did not establish rapport right away; their interactions remained relatively formal and focused throughout her cancer care. When Mary Lee discovered that not only was her physician a big Cubs fan but also had spent time in medical school in Springfield, where she had practiced law for more than thirty-five years, they became more relaxed in conversations with each other.

It is tempting to think of Mary Lee and her oncologists only as individuals and to expect any two individuals to have to negotiate interactions in roughly the same ways. To a great extent, that is true, and we talk more about how individuals affect cancer care in the next chapter. Culture, too, can play an oft-hidden role in healthcare communication, however, as it did between Mary Lee and her physicians. Often, we are not even aware of how our culture shapes our outlooks and responses, our ways of thinking and behaving.

In this chapter, we talk about how to understand culture, apply it to the cancer care situation, and recognize how it may affect decision-making and health care. Because culture is a large topic and because the concepts we cover here are foundational for subsequent chapters, this chapter is one of the lengthier sections of this book.

Culture and the Individual

A person's life experiences and cultural background play a major role in how she or he views, receives, and communicates about health and health care. In the broadest sense, the term *culture* refers to how a community defines, classifies, and represents their experiences. In other words, the beliefs and behaviors of a large group of people—Irish-Americans, senior citizens, or attorneys—underpin that group's community. For an individual, culture can include race, ethnicity, gender, age, religious preferences, income, and educational background. Although we each have diverse physical characteristics and personalities that make us unique, culture provides one method by which a person views and experiences the world as connected with others. Culture provides a way an individual, often unconsciously, sees and experiences affinities and differences between oneself and other individuals. Culture is a way to express ourselves, and we often call these shared expressions *customs*. We create ourselves and present ourselves to others all the time, and we use shared customs, assumptions, and expectations to do that. We create culture via our daily interactions with the world—how we dress, what we eat, how we spend our time—and our daily interactions create the culture in which we live day to day.

Culture shapes values and beliefs about our own health and what health means, as well as shaping our expectations for every visit to a healthcare provider, our knowledge about and attitude toward the healthcare system, and the societal norms about what it means to have cancer. Familial, local, regional, and national cultures all impact health care because they frame—shape how we view and understand—the policies and procedures of the healthcare system. Culture shapes the way in which health communication occurs, even though we may take cultural norms or customs for granted.

In other words, your view of cancer in general, what it means for you to have cancer, what it is like to undergo treatment and survive cancer, and how to talk about cancer with different people in your life are all constructed based on your cultural orientations. *Cross-cultural communication* occurs when a patient and a healthcare provider—or a friend or co-worker—come from different cultural orientations, perhaps different ethnic backgrounds, educational levels, or genders. If each person in the conversation has a different cultural orientation, each may have different beliefs about and behaviors toward cancer, its treatment, and how to discuss it. In cancer care, therefore, it is important to recognize your own cultural perspective and to understand how it is similar to or different than those around you, whether you are the patient, the caregiver, or the healthcare provider.

What We Take for Granted: Societal Views of Cancer and Cancer Care

Individualist and Collectivist Societies

While there are many ways to think about and categorize culture, one method communication researchers use to think about it is by gauging how *individualist* or *collectivist* a society is. An individualistic society like the United States, Australia, or the United Kingdom tends to highly value independence, autonomy, self-reliance, and achievement. South American societies like Panama, Ecuador, and Guatemala, as well as Asian cultures such as Korea and Japan, tend to place great value on social status and groups, including extended families, and are considered collectivist. While commonalities exist across disparate cultures, cultural psychologists sometimes point to contrasts between Eastern (i.e., Asia) and Western (i.e., Western Europe and North America) societies.

These societies can be considered as differing according to how they balance collectivism and individualism. An ongoing or dominant focus on *collectivism* is defined as embeddedness of individuals within social frames that encourages and reinforces *interdependence* among in-group members. Societies that maintain an ongoing or dominant focus on such interdependence are said to be collectivistic. *Individualism* is defined as separation of individuals from social frames that encourages and reinforces *independence* of the self from others. Societies that maintain an ongoing or dominant focus on independence are said to be individualistic. These terms are used most often when discussing comparisons between countries—or other large cultural communities—and assume that differences in levels of individualism and collectivism explain, in part, between-country differences in communication and interaction (Schwarz, Oyserman, & Peytcheva, 2010).

Those individuals grounded in more individualistic-oriented cultures, such as the United States, seem to make fewer adjustments to the ways they communicate when in a different cultural environment than do individuals from more collectivistic-oriented cultures. As an example, Westerners tend to communicate with Taiwanese people using outspoken, terse, or rough spoken language and make few adjustments during the exchanges, according to research based on in-depth interviews, participant observation, and secondary data comparing the cross-cultural communication processes and potential influences of Confucianism and the theory of "manners of different orders" between Easterners and Westerners in Taiwan. On the other hand, Easterners tend to communicate with a more moderate, softer approach and also tend to make adjustments in communication to match more closely the custom of the local culture (Hsieh, 2010).

These distinctions are not absolutes but do offer a range to consider as one thinks about what culture means for a cancer patient. Panama, for example, is not as collectivist a society as Japan but is far less individualist than the United States. Cultures are not either/or so much as on a range that varies from individualistic to collectivistic. Of course, individual people within any society also vary widely in their adherence to cultural norms.

Despite our wonderful uniqueness, these cultural distinctions—individualist and collectivist—nonetheless shape our attitudes and behaviors and also influence the responses others have to our behaviors. A cancer patient in the United States, for instance, may be likely to view her cancer as a personal matter, may resist relying on others for help, and may value having as much control over her own body as possible. Providers in the United States may also reflect the culture's individualistic orientation by being less supportive of healthcare decision-making shared among family members even though a cancer diagnosis affects those family members.

Collectivism describes characteristics of a cultural group that emphasizes needs, vales, objectives, and points of view of an in-group that embody interdependence, field sensitivity, conformity, mutual influence, empathy, sacrifice, and trust of other in-group members (e.g., Hispanic cultures). Individualism, on the other hand, describes characteristics of a cultural group in which members determine social behavior in terms of needs, values, objectives, and points of view that encourage independence, competition, and achievement (e.g., American or German cultures) (Hofstede, 1980; Marin & Triandis, 1985). Further, research indicates that collectivistic cultures prefer interpersonal relationships and in-groups that are nurturing, loving, intimate, and respectful, whereas individualistic cultures prefer superordinate, hierarchical, and confrontational interactions (Triandis, Marin, Hui, Lisansky, & Ottati, 1984). Understanding these preferences and patterns toward interpersonal relationships and preferences for personal contact can be of great importance as healthcare providers within an individualistic-oriented culture interact with more collectivistic-oriented cultures, and vice versa. Awareness and understanding is important because interactions involving distinct cultural and health beliefs may greatly impact the effectiveness of the healthcare encounter.

One difficulty encountered by researchers is that these same collectivistic characteristics and the resulting tendency to shape a gentler or nurturing encounter may lead an individual to give socially desirable responses (Hofstede, 1980). For instance, a phenomenon dubbed *simpatía* acts like a cultural script in which each actor with a collectivistic orientation anticipates the desires or needs of the other in order to meet those desires or needs. The individual tries, often without thinking about it, to create interactions that promote empathy, conformity, and pleasant social relationships and that avoid conflict and negativity. In research situations, simpatía may influence whether an individual who is part of a more collectivistic culture participates in research and also foster high participant completion rates in follow-up interviews. In addition, informal or beside-the-point conversation before and after the formal interview is generally preferred by members of collectivistic-oriented cultures, since it can increase respondent satisfaction and cooperation and build an empathic relationship between the researcher and respondent (Marin & Marin, 1991).

Simpatía is a cultural script that may likewise govern patient–provider interactions. Members of collectivistic-oriented cultures may be more satisfied with healthcare interactions that exhibit empathy, conformity, and pleasant exchanges, including small talk at the beginning and end of an encounter. Providers using such an unseen or even unconscious script, for instance, may couch negative test results in more positive terms. Patients using such an unseen script may not complain about increasingly serious symptoms and may adhere to treatment regimens more strictly.

Familialism. Familialism, or familismo in Hispanic or Latino cultures, is a cultural value exhibited through strong identification with and attachment to families. This valuing of interconnectedness within a family generates strong feelings of reciprocity, loyalty, and solidarity among family members (Marin & Marin, 1991). Ideas about familialism typically span generations and are associated with perceived obligations to provide financial and emotional support within the family; reliance on relatives for financial, emotional, and other help when needed; and the perception that relatives are behavioral and attitudinal reference points throughout one's entire life span (Marin & Marin, 1991). Researchers working with such populations can benefit from developing a strong understanding and respect for the important role of family. Research into the most effective ways to help individuals in familialistic cultures stop smoking, for example, has shown that identifying particular consequences on the family of changing behavior can be a crucial part of overall motivation for behavior change and smoking cessation (Marin, Marin, Perez-Stable, Otero-Sabogal, & Sabogal, 1990).

Likewise, healthcare providers can take into account family-related reasons for behavior change and treatment compliance. By appealing directing the cancer patient's sense of family values as well as introducing small incentives, providers can motivate both cancer patients and their family members to engage in appropriate or beneficial modes of action in response to the diagnosis, condition, and treatment recommendations.

Power Distance. Power distance is defined as a gauge of interpersonal influence or power existing between two individuals and is another important cultural value that differentiates cultural groups (Hofstede, 1980). The idea of power distance is based on the assumption that societies have powerful individuals. Such power or influence results from acquired or inherited characteristics such as education or wealth or from personal traits such as intelligence. In relationships or interactions, individuals often have differing levels of power, or power distance. In such cases, the powerful individual strives to retain that power. In addition, a society as a whole leans toward maintaining existing power differences. Members of low power-distance cultures tend to value and accept interactions that are more democratic and consultative, whereas members of high power-distance cultures tend to value and accept more autocratic, paternalistic, and hierarchical relations.

In considering how power distance affects the provider–patient interaction, one might gauge between the physician, who holds power based on education and expertise, and the patient, who may feel less powerful not only because of lack of expertise relevant to the interaction but also because of physical discomfort or pain. Providers who value a high level of power distance may wear a white coat that symbolizes expertise and use medical terminology and firm tone of voice that convey confidence and authority. Providers who value a low level of power distance may roll up their sleeves, sit at eye level or lower than the patient, and express empathy for the patient's situation. Providers who are attentive to each patient's orientation to power distance can adjust interactions to put the patient at ease with greater or lesser power distance.

Power distance also has important implications in terms of obstacles and access to health information and health care as well. Less powerful individuals in high power-distance cultures, such as the unemployed or those without a college education, tend to face more barriers and fewer access points to health care. This phenomenon likely increases health disparities in terms of entering the healthcare system and in terms of treatment options and benefits.

As Sparks and Miller-Day (2014) consider in their work on health communication and culture, Geert Hofstede's (1980) power distance index (ranging from 1–120) shows higher scores for Latin and Asian countries (sometimes above 90), African areas, and the Arab world. These cultures value high power distance. Anglo and German countries, on the other hand, score lower on the measure of power distance. For instance, Austria = 11, Denmark = 18, and Israel = 13, all very low scores. The United States = 40, United Kingdom = 35, and Sweden = 31 on Hofstede's scale are still low scoring on this index.

When a provider is working with individuals from cultures that value lower power distance, that provider can expect less respect, deference, and consideration of titles, such as M.D. In addition, such patients and caregivers tend to prefer and appreciate informal interaction with more spontaneity, more patient involvement, and joint decision-making about care. Providers working with individuals from cultures who value higher power distance will likely be more effective by offering clear, direct instructions and deadlines. In addition, such situations might call for an authoritarian and research-based approach to treatment, an overt show of respect and deference to those in higher positions, and face-saving responses when dealing with patient disclosure of personal information. Providers and patients comfortable with high power distance may also expect and be less frustrated by the levels of bureaucracy in a healthcare organization.

Personal Space. Preferences for personal and physical space interaction differ from culture to culture as well. Anthropologists have long studied similarities and differences among the ways cultures value space in interactions. Individuals in contact-oriented cultures (e.g., Hispanic or Latino cultures) prefer physical closeness, shorter interpersonal distances, and personal contact. Non-contact-oriented cultures prefer more physical, interpersonal, and personal distance (Hall, 1969). Therefore, providers should be aware that they are navigating physical, interpersonal, and personal space in every interaction with a patient. How a provider establishes affinity and connections with a patient is important to consider as part of cancer care. The first interpersonal encounter, physical examinations and medical procedures that require physical contact, and ongoing communication of various types can benefit when the provider understands each patient's cultural attitudes toward personal space.

Time Orientation. Decades ago, Kluckhohn and Strodbeck (1961) observed that different cultures think about time differently. In other words, individuals in one culture orient themselves to time in certain ways that may not be shared or valued by individuals in other cultures. Some cultures are more future-oriented, and others are more present-oriented. The United States is a future-oriented culture that values and encourages efficiency, planning, and punctuality. Individuals in this culture tend be able to delay gratification. Individuals in present-oriented cultures, on the other hand, are often less invested in arriving on time or meeting deadlines and tend to value a flexible attitude toward time constraints more than efficiency.

Obviously, attitudes toward time can have significant implications for the relationship between provider and patient, especially in the cancer context. Physicians whose work is measured by billable hours may be very aware of the clock and highly efficient. Patients whose cultural attitudes are present oriented may be more patient in the waiting room but also expect more time be spent talking informally during interactions about treatment. Patients who are future-oriented or deadline-oriented may be more conscientious about scheduling regular appointments and adhering to schedules for medication or other treatments than those who are present oriented.

Gender Roles. Over the last several decades, gender roles have shifted, sometimes dramatically, in many societies. Stereotypic perceptions of male and female roles, however, still differ, especially in cultures that are more traditional generally (Marin & Marin, 1991). For instance, men in or from some cultures may be suspicious of a physician of either gender who talks directly with his wife or daughter and may want to be present when female family members interact with the provider. This machismo attitude can have important implications for providers, especially because discussions about cancer diagnosis and treatment can be emotional or sensitive topics for the patient and family. In order to create shared ground, a provider may opt to involve the entire family in sensitive conversations to have a fruitful and productive dialogue for joint decision-making, treatment compliance, and better health outcomes. If traditional gender roles threaten to interfere with treatment, adjustments can help reduce health disparities in the long run, not only for the patient but for other individuals in the family and community who share traditional cultural attitudes about gender.

In all these considerations of cultural variance among patients, one should also consider how physicians, as well as patients, are cultural beings with deeply engrained attitudes in relation to such aspects as power distance, gender, and other attitudes and behaviors. In fact, *gender*—the cultural and social implications of presenting as male or female—plays an important role in medical specialization and compensation. Though it has not always been the case, obstetrics and pediatrics are overwhelmingly female specializations, for instance, whereas radiology is a male-dominated field of medicine (American Medical Association, 2015). Consider also what it means, for example, for medical school faculty salaries to be higher for men than for women, regardless of specialization, experience, or accomplishment (Jena, Olenski, & Blumenthal, 2016). While a physician may be drawn to a field for many reasons, cultural gender roles and expectations also play a part in a physician's professional life and interpersonal interactions.

Taking a Holistic View. Within cultural groups, individuals differ as different identities—national origin, religion and faith preferences, migration and generational history, language use and preferences—intersect. Even among subgroups based on background characteristics, an individual may hold unique cultural values and exhibit behavior that is not considered the norm for that subgroup (Marin & Marin, 1991). One must be attentive to the ways in which culture shapes an individual and the ways in which a person's attitudes and behaviors are connected to the cultural groups and subgroups to which they belong. One must avoid using this approach as an excuse to stereotype and, instead, use this approach to acknowledge and respond to variance among patients and intersecting aspects of each patient's cultural background and position. The information included here can serve as a set of definitional tools to more effectively understand and talk about sensitive cancer issues but is not intended to be prescriptive to individuals or specific scenarios.

A *holistic* view acknowledges that a patient cannot be removed from his or her cultural context or analyzed and treated without taking that context into account. A cancer patient in a more collectivistic society such as Korea or Japan may not feel isolated by cancer and, instead, see the diagnosis as reason for increased family and community cohesion in which the group sacrifices as a whole to ensure the best possible care (Collins, Villagran, & Sparks, 2008). On the other hand, a cancer diagnosis can be a social *stigma*, or social disgrace, for the family or group in countries where it is associated with death and remains *taboo*, or socially prohibited, to speak about. Research indicates that, in Chinese culture, such stigmatizing of cancer may lead all involved—patient, healthcare provider, family member, caregiver—to resist, perhaps unconsciously, sharing information with each other (Mok & Martinson, 2000). Some Chinese and Latino caregivers may be encultured to not seek information from others for fear of disclosing the patient's cancer diagnosis or current distress (Collins et al., 2008; Mok & Martinson, 2000). In order to avoid conflict and be polite, a patient from or within certain communities may give incomplete or not completely honest answers to questions perceived to be embarrassing and may pursue treatment recommendations without fully considering one's own preferences. These cultural and individual preferences introduce challenges to creating shared meaning between providers and patients. An awareness of these challenges allows them to be addressed through communication.

For different reasons—in different cultures or based on different life experiences—cancer patients view issues of privacy differently and may withhold information from healthcare providers that could change the options and recommendations for treatment (Petronio, 2002). A person with lung cancer, for instance, may not tell his physician that he is still smoking. The withholding of such information may stem from a sense of autonomy—it is none of your business—in a society like Australia or from a sense of being punished for an unbalanced lifestyle in a society like China. A person with nausea after chemotherapy treatment may minimize the seriousness of the symptoms, either because he wants to be strong enough to handle it on his own or because he wants to hide his suffering from others who might be affected by it. Patients who are aware of their attitudes and providers who understand a range of attitudes among patients, as well as their own attitudes as physicians, can work together toward shared meaning and understanding of specific situations and options

In her book, Robin Roberts (2014) discussed openly feelings that many patients keep hidden, including that she sometimes felt embarrassed to have a serious illness. She wondered why she had developed cancer, especially because she thought of herself as athletic and taking good care of her health. She wondered whether she had done something that had caused her cancer and whether others would assume that she had done something wrong or not taken care of herself appropriately. Dealing with a health issue, such as cancer, changes the boundaries for communication in close relationships, as disclosing illness may make individuals feel embarrassed, uncomfortable, or exposed (Petronio, 2002).

It is not clear where Roberts picked up those ideas, but that attitude echoes Patricia Grace King's initial response—surprise, why me?—to her cancer diagnosis. That is a response that reflects individualistic values such as self-reliance. Considering your feelings and how your background and interactions shape those feelings can be an important step in improving your communication with others about cancer, whether you are a patient or a provider.

Individualism in Action

Sally Ride, the first American woman in space, was exceptionally competitive and private, hallmarks of someone in an individualistic society. An individualistic attitude, along with a lot of knowledge and drive, probably helps a person like Ride become an astronaut, and those qualities are admired in the United States.

When she was diagnosed with pancreatic cancer, Ride kept that news a secret from the public, just as she had her decades-long relationship with her life partner Tam O'Shaughnessy. Ride's secret-keeping seemed to be driven by what researchers have defined as a strong sense of professionalism and a view of privacy management (Petronio, 2002). In addition, as Lynn Sherr (2014) documents in her biography of the astronaut, Ride's decisions may also have resulted from fears of culturally based reactions the American public has about physical weakness and about sexual orientation. Perhaps she wanted to be remembered as young, strong, and smiling, as she existed in those iconic photos taken aboard the space shuttle. Sally Ride saw herself, in part, as others saw her: a symbol for ambitious young girls and for NASA and space exploration. As Sherr (2014) wrote in Ride's biography, Ride was concerned that she would be treated differently, so she employed privacy and carefully managed her own levels of disclosure, which is a response also borne out by research (Petronio, 2002).

In *A Real Emotional Girl*, Tanya Chernov (2012) wrote about her father, who was diagnosed with colorectal cancer. Like Sally Ride, he had not shared his diagnosis very widely and remained very private, in part because he ran a summer camp for kids and was a strong, vibrant father figure to those campers and their families. Like Ride, he saw himself, in part, as others saw him, as a symbol as well as an individual. He wanted to maintain that fatherly leadership role and not burden others with the news.

Chernov (2012) waited for her father to complain about the pain he experienced from his cancer, the surgeries, and the chemotherapy and radiation. "My dad often spoke of his pre- and post-cancer pain thresholds—how 'cancer pain' seemed to exist on a whole other scale" (p. 97), she wrote. But he only rarely whispered to his wife that he did not feel very well and, even with a tube down his nose and with body soreness from radiation, he never complained to his daughter. Chernov (2012) wrote: "His strength and resilience were a testament to how much he loved his family and how much he loved life—he just kept on going without drawing attention to his discomfort because he wanted to be here with us so badly and wanted to make the most of our time together to the very extent of his diminishing ability" (p. 97). While her father wanted to live as long as he could to be with his family, he seemed to approach his illness as an individual burden, not one easily shared by his family or larger community. Her father's attitude epitomizes the values of the individualistic culture in which he lived and also his position in society as a strong, loving leader.

Robin Roberts, the television host, recounts a different kind of individualism in action, one that can have serious consequences: *noncompliance*, or not following the directions of your healthcare provider. Roberts (2014) admits, "I wasn't taking all the prescribed medications I should have been taking. I got a little cocky, felt I was doing okay and didn't want to take some of the medications" (p. 238). Her admission came when she faced a health crisis during her recovery and then looked to her own behavior as a possible obstacle in her recovery. Whether it is taking medication exactly as directed or avoiding exposure to germs that might cause infection, patients must beware of their urge to take health matters completely into their own hands. Providers, likewise, must understand that cultural attitudes, such as those emerging from individualistic or collectivistic cultural contexts, affect patient behavior.

Collectivism and Individualism in Cancer Care

Family members in collectivistic cultures are more likely to be involved and play a major role in cancer care for a loved one. Several family members may attend doctor visits with a parent or grandparent, and the patient and family may expect group discussion and decision-making. In an effort to allow a cancer patient to save face and avoid being forced to talk about cancer, some families may prefer to communicate directly with the physician without the patient present and to bear the burden of the illness themselves instead of having the patient bear the burden.

Providers in the United States often expect patients to make decisions about treatment options relatively quickly, but this can lead to problems, especially for individuals from collectivistic cultures. This approach can be challenging for the patient and for family members involved in the decision-making who want to discuss options together. A Hmong patient, for example, may harbor culturally based mistrust or language-based misunderstanding and may want to consult an older family member or a high-status male family member for advice, and other family members may be hesitant to make a decision about healthcare treatment for a family member without consulting this person (Johnson, 2002). In Japan, providers often do not tell a patient about the terminal cancer diagnosis (Kakai, 2002), sometimes allowing informed family members to make treatment decisions. Japanese physicians have begun to share this sort of health information with patients more regularly, and the majority of Japanese patients indicate that, if they have cancer, they want to be informed by their physicians of their condition (Long, 2000). Many Japanese individuals, however, prefer ambiguous communication from a physician about a cancer diagnosis (Kakai, 2002) to decrease distress and allow family members to remain hopeful about a loved one's recovery instead of viewing the diagnosis as the end of life.

Gudykunst and colleagues examined the influence of individualism–collectivism on communication within in-group (I belong) and out-group (I do not belong) relationships and found significant differences between in-group and out-group communication in collectivistic cultures as evidenced by self-monitoring and predicted-outcome value of the relationships. The distinction a person makes between those groups to which one belongs and those groups with which one does not associate affects communication processes in interpersonal relationships. Results based on data collected from 850 college students in Hong Kong and Japan (collectivistic) and in Australia and the United States (individualistic) suggest that members of collectivistic cultures draw sharper divisions between in-group and out-group than do members of individualistic cultures (Gudykunst et al., 1992). This research suggests that, for some individuals, attitudes and behaviors that distinguish them as not belonging to particular groups may be as important as and intertwined with attitudes and behaviors that demonstrate affiliation with an in-group. Withholding a diagnosis from a patient may be perceived as a way that the patient can maintain the out-group status, thereby avoiding the label of a person with cancer.

In the United States, this practice of keeping the diagnosis or treatment information from the patient goes directly against the standard practices and rules about informed consent. Cancer care providers in individualistic countries that value autonomy and self-reliance may not agree to honor a decision to conceal a diagnosis or withhold medical information from the patient, even if it is common practice in the patient's home country, community, or culture. Patients in the United States must be informed about their condition and cancer treatment protocols so that they can make the choice whether to pursue specific treatment options.

Consensual and Top-Down Decisions

Cultural and individual differences can lead to different kinds of decision-making. In her book *The Culture Map*, Erin Meyer (2014) discusses two different approaches to decision-making in the business world: *consensual* and *top-down*. When consensus is a vital aspect of the decision-making process, as it tends to be in German businesses, it may take a while to make the decision. "But once that decision has been made," she writes, "the implementation is quite rapid, since everyone has completely bought in and the decision is fixed and inflexible" (p. 149). When the decision rests with an individual, as is often the case in U.S.-based businesses, "decisions tend to be made quickly, early in the process, by one person (likely the boss). But each decision is also flexible" (p. 149).

Consider how these cultural differences in the decision-making process might apply to a cancer patient. Do you expect to take your time making a decision about the next step in your treatment, in part so that you can gather both information and opinions to build consensus among your healthcare team, your family, and yourself? Or do you expect to make decisions about your health care quickly yourself, with the ability to adjust the decision as you gather more information or circumstances change? Or do you expect your healthcare provider to make decisions about your treatment? What Meyer (2014) says about the business world applies to health care as well: "Either of these systems can work, as long as everyone understands and follows the rules of the game" (p. 149).

Who Is Really in Charge? Interpersonal Dynamics in Cancer Care

Cultural context always informs the relationship between the patient and the healthcare provider, though sometimes in subtle or unnoticed ways. Many cultures place great emphasis on respect for persons in positions of power, and physicians are usually perceived as being in positions of power. When a patient has cancer and the doctor can provide treatment, the doctor has a certain kind of power that affects all the interpersonal interactions they have. In addition, a person who is feeling unwell or worried may feel more lacking in power than is normally the case for that individual.

Think about a specific scenario between a physician and a cancer patient. A doctor is likely to tell a patient, "Make an appointment to see me again if you feel any more pain. Don't wait for it to worsen before you come in." It is unlikely, on the other hand that the patient, even if exhausted and in pain, would respond, "Next time I come for an appointment, I don't want you to leave me in the waiting room for over an hour before I see you." Even though the exchange seems honest and clear, the first example would likely be viewed as a reasonable instruction, whereas the second statement would be viewed—by both provider and patient—as unusual and perhaps inappropriate. Even using the command verbs *make* and *don't wait* instead of couching the request in phrasing such as *I want (or don't want)* indicates a difference in each person's position in the relationship.

Likewise, it is common for a physician to address patients by first name, whereas it is uncommon for a person to turn the tables. In the situation that opens this chapter, Dr. Malhotra called Mary Lee *Mary*, despite her two-part name, which became a little joke over time, but Mary Lee never called him *Rajat*. Even more striking is that the physician is likely to expect to touch and probe the patient's body, whereas a patient is not likely to initiate physical contact. Imagine a patient asking one's physician to step onto the scale or reveal weekly alcohol consumption. The situation does not allow for that exchange of information—or exchanging that sort of information in both directions. That exchange does not make sense in the context of cancer care because of engrained cultural assumptions and expectations and also because the focus is on the biomedical situation of the patient. Turning the tables disrupts cultural norms and individual expectations. In fact, sometimes we notice cultural norms only when they are disrupted. That difference between what is appropriate behavior and communication for a healthcare provider and what is appropriate or comfortable for a patient displays the seemingly natural power difference between the provider and patient.

Power differences often go unnoticed because individuals tend to meet cultural expectations for a given interaction. This patient–provider power difference can work in positive ways because matching cultural expectations may be less stressful than bucking customs and roles. This power difference sometimes, however, can lead to undesired outcomes for cancer patients and their families. Patients from communities that place a great emphasis on status, for instance, may ask fewer questions of their physicians in medical conversations because the patient is concerned about challenging the doctor's authority and does not want to be perceived as disrespectful. Despite a strong desire for information, patients and their families may resist asking questions they think might be viewed either as difficult for the physician to answer or as trivial. Providers who highly value status may perceive difficult questions as meant to reveal weakness, whereas trivial questions might be thought of as wasting the provider's valuable time. While a rushed provider may have run into a scheduling snafu that day, a physician rushing through medical conversations with a patient can sometimes be driven by cultural norms.

Because providers are experts and hold a position of authority in conversations with patients about cancer, they are often comfortable controlling medical interactions and dictating the relationships they have with patients. Patients need information but how that information is conveyed is also important in shaping the relationship, including the patient's comfort conversing openly. Regardless of cultural differences, patients need comfort, affiliation, and respect from providers. We discuss patient–provider communication further and how to foster comfort, affiliation, and respect in interactions and decision-making during cancer care in Chapter 7.

Culture and Patient Attitudes

Culturally Based Reasoning

Consider the different ways you figure things out and learn. Did you learn math by grasping the concepts—the general principles—first and then applying them? Many people in Italy, Germany, and Mexico had this kind of education. Did you learn a foreign language by beginning with grammatical structures and vocabulary? Again, that is what Erin Meyer (2014), in *The Culture Map*, calls *principles-first reasoning*. But you may have learned a foreign language in a different way, by walking into the classroom and being bombarded by questions in the language you did not yet understand. That is called *applications-first reasoning*.

Most people use both kinds of reasoning, but your background can lead you to prefer or depend on one more than the other. When it comes to cancer care, the important thing to remember is that using principles-first learning tends to lead us to focus on *why* something has happened or is recommended, whereas using applications-first learning tends to lead us to focus on *how* something has happened or will be accomplished. If we apply the ideas from Meyer (2014), we can surmise that people raised in Australia, Canada, and the United States tend to use applications-first learning and, therefore, focus more on *how*, on the process, rather than on *why*, the reasons. That cultural context may make such patients, for example, more interested in hearing what treatment their physicians propose and what they need to do next than in hearing background information about their own situation or about the reasons for pursuing one treatment instead of another.

Fatalism and Cancer

A person's culture and life experiences can greatly influence one's attitude toward cancer. Some people think, *If someone is meant to get cancer, he will.* This attitude is often referred to as *fatalism*, which means that the person believes fate plays a large role in what happens to him. (It does not mean that the person believes cancer is fatal.) Fatalistic views of cancer may be influenced by racial, ethnic, religious, educational, and/or socioeconomic history. In a positive sense, fatalism can lead some cancer patients toward accepting the difficult diagnosis or can aid patients in not blaming themselves for getting cancer. But fatalism can also lead a patient down the path of feeling powerless to get well. Unfortunately, this attitude can keep patients from being active in their health care, as if nothing they can do will change the outcome (Sparks & Villagran, 2008).

Religious beliefs can shape patients' attitudes toward fatalism in different ways. Certainly, for cancer patients and their families, religious beliefs can offer ways to generate or sustain hope. Religious convictions can also include a belief that God, or some other higher power, ultimately holds power over who gets cancer and whether that person will recover. Research suggests that many Latinos with strong religious beliefs, for instance, may believe an illness such as cancer is predestined or handed down by God, in which case the patient may feel that the disease should be accepted or endured as part of fulfilling

God's will (Sparks & Villagran, 2008, 2010). In these cases, a patient and family members may view treatment (or lack of treatment) as God's overall plan. Patients and family members with these personal beliefs tend to handle distress well. They also may resist a provider's treatment recommendations and may hesitate to follow up with questions about treatment. Providers who remain unaware of such cultural attitudes may become frustrated by their patients' resistance. Understanding a patient's attitude toward fatalism can be fostered by and can foster strong communication about cancer and treatment.

Beliefs in Life After Death

What a patient believes about life after death also influences the way that patient views one's own cancer, treatment, and prognosis. These beliefs are especially important for patients and providers to consider when cancer is in an advanced stage, prognosis is poor, or treatment options are limited. Providers who work with *terminally ill* cancer patients—those who are expected to die from the illness—should be very respectful about the patient's attitudes about life after death. Patients who have similar beliefs as their providers might find comfort in talking about religious issues or engaging in religious activities such as praying together. Or they may seek additional guidance from someone who shares their beliefs, perhaps a priest or rabbi. Many hospitals and hospice care services offer spiritual counseling because of its recognized importance in overall well-being. Whether the patient is Buddhist, Christian, Jewish, Muslim, Hindu, Atheist, part of another religious culture, or not religious at all, a provider who comes from a different background from a particular patient must find ways to communicate in a manner that shows respect for that patient's religious convictions or absence of religious convictions. Likewise, a patient whose emotional or spiritual needs extend beyond the provider's familiarity or comfort may want to focus entirely on biomedical information with the provider and may seek other types of support elsewhere. In fact, we discuss this issue further in Chapter 7.

Respect should not be confused, though, with making false assumptions about individuals from other communities. Open, clear communication between the patient and the provider can dispel assumptions so that the patient can make the best decisions. Those whose beliefs differ from their provider should be especially cognizant of asking about the outcomes—expected improvements, risks, side effects—for specific recommended treatments so that they can consider the medical information in relation to their own beliefs and attitudes.

The Language Barrier and Learning the Lingo

Almost all cancer patients are faced with the challenge of learning new terminology, so language is an issue that applies to communication across the board in cancer care. For instance, when television host Robin Roberts (2014) was diagnosed with myelodysplastic syndrome, the specialist called to say that she had MDS. Because she had never heard of MDS, she thought he was telling her that she had MS, or multiple sclerosis. Because she started asking questions, her confusion was quickly addressed, and she came to understand that she had a condition in her blood that had resulted from her earlier, successful treatment for breast cancer and that would, if left untreated, develop into cancer. Questions, even if they repeat information you have just heard, are often the best way to ensure any overt or hidden confusion is corrected quickly.

Even when the provider and patient share a primary language, regional or national differences in the use of that language can impact the meaning of communication. Terminology related to cancer care in Great Britain may be different from terms used in the United States, even though English is the primary language in both countries. Even in the United States, phrasing by someone from the Deep South may differ from that of a person from the Northeast. The healthcare system can be a confusing maze of information for anyone diagnosed with cancer but especially when materials—brochures or websites, for example—cross cultures or languages, as many people may not consider the cultural and linguistic difficulties of translation.

Even if patient and provider share communities and languages, the patient is unlikely to have in-depth knowledge of medicine and cancer. In addition to the actual words spoken by patients and healthcare providers, how the words are used provides clues to their meaning, and these nuances are culturally bound. In other words, choices to say or not say certain things, as well as the stress put on certain words or syllables, can change the meaning of a message. One person may use the word *nausea* to describe occasional indigestion, for instance, whereas another may use the same word to describe ongoing vomiting but not mild intestinal discomfort. If a patient says something like, *I can only walk to church*, does that person mean that driving has become impossible, that a farther walk has become impossible, or that more frequent exercise is no longer possible? As this example illustrates, even a patient and provider who are talking in the same language can miss the real meaning of a message even when they understood the other person's words.

When a patient and one's physician, nurse, or technician do not share a common primary language, miscommunication is more likely to occur, and patients may become exhausted just making sure they understand what to do next, let alone doing it. Language barriers impede access to health organizations, diminish the potential quality of healthcare services, and increase the risk of unintended health outcomes or mistakes.

Healthcare facilities are often required or opt to provide translators for patients whose primary language differs from that spoken by the provider. However, translators usually play a limited role in patient care and decision-making, a patient may not have the same translator throughout care, and many translators have little experience translating information about cancer care specifically. Moreover, language barriers can impact the most basic needs for patients, including finding appropriate healthcare facilities, scheduling appointments, reading signage in medical facilities, completing patient medical histories and other forms, and reading prescription information, including that about drug interaction. Translation of information is often confusing because the translations do not always convey the intended meaning of what is written or said. In fact, the same combination of words in two different languages may have two different meanings. It is one thing to not understand something that has been said, but it may be worse to think you understand something you have been told when you are unknowingly wrong. In that case, a patient or a family member may not even realize that it would be important to ask clarification questions.

In some instances, family members who attend doctor visits can translate information, which can be helpful in ensuring clear provider–patient communication. Even though family members may have strong skills in both languages, family members often are not experienced in a healthcare environment, may struggle to interpret medical jargon, or may make missteps when relaying treatment options or drug protocols. Especially when translating sensitive information, family members can impede open communication between patients and providers when neither the patient nor the family member wants to feel embarrassment. Physicians may hesitate to ask sensitive questions in the presence of the patient's family members. Patients, too, may withhold sensitive information in the presence of family. Latino men, for example, are less likely during a screening for testicular cancer to share full information about their symptoms when a family member is in the room (Sparks & Villagran, 2008). The person who is the best translator may not be the person with whom the patient is most comfortable sharing information.

The most serious language barriers are often the easiest to notice and, therefore, can often be readily addressed. That is a good thing. Other cultural differences and assumptions may be less obvious and, therefore, remain hidden and unaddressed.

Gender and Cancer Care

Biological *sex*—the biological, anatomical, or genetic distinction between male and female—and the physical body that comes with such distinction account for some differences in cancer incidence and mortality rates. It is true, for example, that females are far more likely to get breast cancer than males because of biological differences. Because they don't have testicles, females do not get testicular cancer. Likewise, males are not diagnosed with ovarian or uterine cancer. Of course, it is possible for an intersex patient who has internal female reproductive organs as well as external male genitals to develop cancer in any of those areas.

In addition to biological differences, gender differences and related cultural patterns are also important. Men are statistically more likely to get lung cancer, for instance, yet some of the reasons are based in gender not biological differences. Men historically have been more likely than women to work in occupations that expose them to *carcinogens*—substances known to potentially cause cancer—such as insecticides, pesticides, and diesel. For decades, those who identify as men were also more likely to smoke cigarettes. Smoking became glamorous for women in the United States in the middle of the last century, however, and women are also more likely to smoke as a means to control their weight because there are stronger social pressures on women than on men to be thin. As a result, women are catching up with lung cancer. As Siddhartha Mukherjee (2010) puts it in his book *The Emperor of All Maladies*,

> Death rates [from lung cancer] among men had peaked and dropped off by the mid-1980s. In contrast, lung cancer mortality had dramatically risen in women, particularly in older women, and it was still rising. Between 1970 and 1994, lung cancer deaths among women over the age of fifty-five had increased by 400 percent, more than the rise in the rates of breast and colon cancer *combined*. (p. 331)

Differences between men and women in rates of lung cancer, therefore, can be traced to gender norms that are culturally constructed, rather than being solely biologically based.

Within a culture, men and women have different roles and ranges of behaviors that tend to be most acceptable. The World Health Organization (2007), in a report on gender equity, states that gender is a powerful social determinant of health that interacts with other important factors, such as a patient's age, family structure, income, education, and social support. (We talk more about how age affects cancer care in Chapter 5.) One study (Malmusi, Artazcoz, Benach, & Borell, 2011) indicated that women in Spain were more likely to report being in ill health than men as a result of actual higher disease burden, especially conditions associated with chronic pain, but not necessarily higher mortality. A different study (Din et al., 2015) in the United Kingdom found that, for six cancers, the time between developing symptoms and diagnosis was longer for women.

Because early diagnosis is often associated with higher five-year survival rates and a wider range of effective treatment options, potential gender inequity is important to consider early in the cancer care continuum. Are women less likely to seek out and report symptoms to a healthcare provider? Are women less likely to talk about their symptoms in ways that providers take seriously or interpret as a serious risk to health? Do providers tend to take reports of ill health more seriously from male patients? Do providers take into account gender differences in conversational styles when talking with patients about symptoms? How can providers help the patient live the best life possible, regardless of biological sex and gender identification?

As another example of how important gender is in cancer care, consider Robin Roberts's (2014) reminder: "Breast cancer is the number one killer of women in the UAE [United Arab Emirates]. Many succumb because the stigma surrounding the disease in that part of the world prevents them from seeking early detection" (p. 53). When it is caught early, breast cancer is almost always treatable and the patient is likely to remain cancer free after treatment. So, the UAE offers a stark example of how social expectations related to gender can jeopardize lives.

While that example is extreme, more subtle social expectations can affect the exchange of information, approaches to decision-making, and cancer care. Gender norms are closely tied to culture, so patients and healthcare providers need to keep these differences among patients in mind. In addition, cross-cultural communication between men and women from different cultures may be especially difficult unless both parties understand the cultural influence of gender on communication.

Healthcare providers who understand cultural gender norms in a particular culture can ask questions appropriate for the patient and offer information to guide that patient. In some communities, the activities of each gender are kept so separate that a patient would find it inappropriate to see a physician of the opposite gender. Some cultures also have strict dress codes for women, for instance, and physical examinations can be stressful or problematic for women who abide by some types of cultural gender norms. Respect for such cultural differences should be extended by the provider, who may limit exposure only to necessary body parts for examination. Providers who share or work to understand the important role of cultural traditions can be more attentive and responsive to their patients' preferences related to gender without compromising good cancer care.

Healthcare providers are becoming more cognizant that the traditional gender and family roles of father, mother, and children are far from adequate in describing all individuals. A patient's sexual orientation, for instance, may be relevant to the patient's physical and emotional well-being during cancer care. In her book *Malignant*, S. Lochlann Jain (2013) points to relatively recent studies that revealed disturbing information about how gay and lesbian patients are treated. "One study," she reports, "found that nearly 80 percent of nurses did not want to touch their gay and lesbian patients" (p. 39). She asserts that lesbians may be likely to receive substandard care, though she also points out that Black women are especially at risk of receiving substandard care (p. 40). These are cultural, in addition to medical, issues, and they must be addressed through literacy and communication—as well as through policy—that allow all individuals to receive the best health care possible and make the best health decisions they can for themselves.

Transgender patients may face specific communication challenges as they negotiate their cancer care. Medicine necessarily focuses on the biological body. For instance, a transgender patient may have a body that does not match the person's gender identity, roles, and pronouns. Unfortunately, physicians rarely receive training that takes distinct needs of transgender patients into account. Every physician should respect each patient's gender, including using the pronouns by which the patient wants to be referred. In considering both biological sex and cultural gender in recommending treatment options, the physician will need to treat the person's anatomy while not determining the patient's social identity by that anatomy.

Building a strong patient–provider relationship, which we discuss at greater length in Chapter 7, allows for a range of relevant information to be shared, for misguided cultural assumptions to be corrected, and for each patient to be viewed as an individual.

Bridging Cultural Gaps

A variety of cultural circumstances may work against an individual's ability to communicate openly and clearly with healthcare providers. Health literacy correlates with economic status and educational status, with populations demonstrating the lowest levels of health literacy likely to be poorer and less educated than populations with higher levels health literacy (Kreps, Neuhauser, Sparks, & Villagran, 2008; Kreps & Sparks, 2008). In other words, a cancer patient's socio-economic status and access to information, facilities, and treatment are related. Lack of access can lead to poor health literacy, and vice versa. As we have discussed, strong provider–patient communication often benefits from high health literacy. Patients and informal caregivers from populations with low levels of health literacy are sometimes confused or misinformed about cancer prevention practices, early cancer detection guidelines, healthcare services, cancer treatment strategies, and the recommended use of medications, which, in turn, can lead to errors and consequences affecting the patient's health (Sparks, 2013). Communities must work against barriers tied to geography, class, race, gender, and other cultural factors.

Healthcare providers may assume a higher level of health literacy generally than they did years ago because the Internet makes health information widely available. However, better-educated adults are much more likely to search for information on the Internet than those with less education (Kreps et al., 2008; Kreps & Sparks, 2008). In addition, now that a great deal of reliable information about cancer is online and many healthcare facilities have extensive websites, lack of access to and ease with using computers can make it difficult for a person to increase one's health literacy and negotiate cancer care. Cancer patients who do not have access to a computer or other device and wifi may not be as prepared for discussions with healthcare providers about tests and treatment as patients who have easy access to online resources. Healthcare providers should discuss with the patient what information that patient already has and how that patient can gather more information. Also, patients should ask for more information whenever they feel healthcare providers are assuming they have more information than they have had the opportunity to gather yet.

Significant differences in the incidence of some diseases and the mortality rate associated with those diseases exist from community to community. Specific underserved cultural groups fare less well when it comes to healthiness, as compared with the health status of the general population (Kreps et al., 2008; Kreps & Sparks, 2008). Pain tolerance and management may even be grounded in cultural differences in ways not fully understood. All patients in pain or with cancer should be treated with equal attention and care, regardless of their race, gender, education, or socio-economic status.

Research consistently indicates that preventative cancer screening rates can be greatly impacted by low health literacy, and communication plays an important role (Kreps et al., 2008). In determining the association between health literacy, communication habits, and colorectal cancer (CRC) screening among low-income patients, researchers found that limited health literacy is a potential barrier to CRC screening. Less than ideal screening rates for CRC were reported among those who had completed less education, so it seems likely that limited health literacy affects some populations' access to or use of cancer detection (Ojinnaka et al., 2015).

More research into the relationships among socio-economic status, education, health literacy, and cancer screening rates are needed to more fully understand the role that health communication can play and how other cultural attitudes may affect access to information about cancer screening as well as access to screening itself. Cancer is the leading cause of death, for instance, among Asian-Americans; the Asian-American population is expected to increase over the next few decades; and Chinese-Americans make up the largest ethnic group among Asian-Americans. Other studies, on the other hand, indicate that low health literacy is associated with lower cancer screening rates but that Asian-American populations tend to have high socio-economic standing and educational attainment rates. Our understanding of cancer prevention and detection among Chinese-American individuals is, therefore, lacking. Despite acknowledgment by the White House of lack of data, this association has not yet been studied in Chinese-American communities specifically (Sentell, Tsoh, Davis, Davis, & Braun, 2015).

Further, a recent study by Sentell et al. (2013) of Hawaiian and Filipino women revealed many health information challenges related to literacy, both in written and oral health communication. Practical challenges included so-called big words, complexity of terms, and lack of plain English. Interpersonal challenges included doctors rushing, doctors not assessing comprehension, and doctors treating respondents as biological bodies not as people. Women noted that they would often not ask questions even when they knew they did not understand information because they did not want the provider to think negatively of them. As a result, the researchers suggest several areas to analyze more fully in order to address gaps in cancer communication: (1) the often crucial role of family and community in the dissemination of health information, (2) the pivotal role women often play in sharing and interpreting health information for others, (3) the relevance of personal experience and interpersonal relationships to how health information is made meaningful for an individual, and (4) the importance of local cultural relevance in health communication (Sentell, Dela Cruz, Heo, & Braun, 2013).

Researchers examining and comparing cancer-related conversations in online forums hosted by Canadian and American associations for retired persons found that health literacy is a crucial component for full engagement and use of online resources and information gathering, particularly for older adults (Donelle & Hoffman-Goetz, 2009). This interaction suggests a circular effect in which increased literacy helps one gather and use information and gathering and using information helps one become more health literate.

Differences in health literacy, access to health care, and fair treatment during diagnosis and treatment often occur, in part, because of bias, prejudice, and stereotyping and because of a lack of communication about health issues within and across communities. *Bias* refers to the tendency to make judgments on preconceived, often deeply embedded, ideas. All people have biases based on their experiences, values, and attitudes, and an individual may find it helpful to think about ways in which preconceived ideas affect the ways we interact and make decisions. *Prejudice* refers to making a judgment without adequate knowledge. Prejudice, therefore, can make us less open to options and more dismissive of other individuals based on characteristics they share with a group. *Stereotyping* is particularly problematic in health communication because it is the application of a popular but often misinformed belief about a group to an individual within that group. To reduce disparities based on bias, prejudice, and stereotyping, we must understand how culture impacts our attitudes, beliefs, and behaviors related to health and health care. This means both gaining a clearer understanding of the impact of culture on patients and also how culture shapes communication among healthcare providers and health organizations responsible for the delivery of medical services.

Not every other person behaves, thinks, or feels exactly like every other individual. When a healthcare professional does not understand actions of patients, their families, or healthcare co-workers, that lack of understanding may be related to cultural beliefs or practice. If healthcare providers and organizations become aware of the different cultural groups and individuals that they may encounter, they can adjust their behaviors during interactions and address discomfort or confusion before that affects a patient's care. The following approaches can help make provider–patient interactions more effective in cancer care.

- Healthcare providers can take cues from the patient and family. When discomfort is sensed during an interaction, the issue might be addressed by briefly explaining one's own assumptions. For instance, a physician might say, "I usually look people in the eyes when I am discussing serious matters, but I understand that not everyone finds that respectful." Bringing assumptions to the foreground encourages empathy, or the understanding of the other's situation.
- Questions encourage others to respond. Since most people do not want to hear bad news, it is sometimes helpful for healthcare providers to preface the details by saying something like, "I know it is difficult to hear bad news, but it is my job to make sure you understand your situation so that you can make the best decisions. Are you ready to discuss the biopsy results?" Even if the other person chooses not to answer questions directly, a back-and-forth can allow both participants in the interaction to receive information and adjust behaviors.
- In the United States, a physician's obligation is to the individual patient, but the patient may want to include others, including individuals outside the family, in decision-making. Seeking additional advice may be only part of a patient's concern. Taking time to talk with others also may help the patient process and analyze information and options.
- Healthcare providers are trained to prevent, diagnose, and treat illnesses, so it may be especially difficult for them when a patient refuses care, especially if that care seems routine or not risky. Patient consent remains necessary, and patients must make decisions about their own care. Only in rare cases, in which the court intervenes on the behalf of a minor, for instance, can physicians treat patients without their consent. Cancer care can be undermined when the assumptions

and goals of the treating physician and the patient are at odds. It is important for the physician to convey the medical information, acknowledge that decisions about treatment are the patient's, discuss assumptions, and work toward shared goals.

- Healthcare providers and organizations should do what they can to make allowances for family members to be with the patient as much as possible. Hospitals are increasingly aware of the positive effects of family support, and some now allow for family to come and go at any hour and even spend the night. For patients who do not have family visiting, the hospital staff may suggest hospital-based programs such as pastoral care or a therapy dog.
- If regular prayer or religious observance is important for a patient, the healthcare provider or organization should try to incorporate these activities into the patient's care and arrange the privacy necessary.
- In general, healthcare providers and organizations want patients to be as comfortable as possible. A patient may benefit from receiving cards and flowers, but some patients, for instance those with compromised immune systems, may have restrictions on items in the room or on visitors. Advising the family to keep valuable items at home is reasonable advice. Whenever possible, the patient should be able to keep personal items at the hospital bedside.

Understanding Culture to Improve Cancer Care

This chapter has revealed some of what cancer communication experts have discovered about how to tailor approaches to cancer care and communication by accounting for the cultural contexts of different individuals so that cancer care can be improved for the individual and for the community. New treatments, equipment, and medications are expensive to develop, and it is good that money is spent on that research. Improving cancer communication among individuals from different cultural backgrounds also has the potential to improve cancer care and survival rate in additional, cost effective ways.

Even more importantly, each individual—patient, caregiver, provider—can use this chapter to strengthen communication right now. For a patient, one's own beliefs about and attitudes toward cancer can sometimes be at odds with the beliefs and approaches of others who are providing information, support, and treatment. Effective communication that emerges from awareness of how culture shapes individual beliefs can help a person negotiate the healthcare system and the various conversations that a patients wants and needs to have about one's cancer. For all individuals involved in the cancer continuum, understanding the role that cultural context plays can help create shared meaning and strong communication.

Exercise & Discussion

Scholars and students in health communication should realize that not every individual in a given interaction shares the same background and cultural assumptions. This classroom activity is designed help students explore their own cultural assumptions and consider how the behaviors of each individual in a healthcare interaction are shaped by cultural frameworks.

Consider and discuss the following examples of cultural beliefs and how healthcare professionals might best address them:

1. People from some cultures tend to believe it is disrespectful to look someone in the eyes while speaking. However, in other cultures, failing to look a person in the eye can be considered a sign of not being honest.
2. People from some cultures tend to prefer to buffer bad news to boost the spirits of the ill person.
3. In some religions, it is important to include the elders of the church in any major decisions that need to be made.
4. Some cultures and religions oppose routine vaccinations and immunization or some kinds of invasive treatment.
5. Family involvement is very important in some cultures. Some patients will have large, close-knit families. Other patients may have no close relatives or no family in close proximity.
6. Some people with religious beliefs may wish to pray five times per day. Others may wish to receive communion weekly.
7. There may be some articles of clothing, religious medals, holy pictures, icons, or other objects that are important to a patient.

References

American Medical Association. (2015). How medical specialties vary by gender. Retrieved from http://www.ama-assn.org/ama/ama-wire/post/medical-specialties-vary-gender

Chernov, T. (2012). *A real emotional girl: A memoir of love and loss*. New York, NY: Skyhorse.

Collins, D., Villagran, M. M., & Sparks, L. (2008). Crossing borders, crossing cultures: Barriers to cancer prevention and treatment along the U.S./Mexico border. *Patient Education and Counseling, 71*, 333–339.

Din, N. U., Ukoumunne, O. C., Rubin, G., Hamilton, W., Carter, B., Stapley, S., Neal, R. D. (2015, May 15). Age and gender variations in cancer diagnostic intervals in 15 cancers: Analysis of data from the UK clinical practice research datalink. *Plos One*. doi:10.1371/journal.pone.0127717

Donelle, L., & Hoffman-Goetz, L. (2009). Functional health literacy and cancer care conversations in online forums for retired persons. *Informatics for Health and Social Care, 34(1)*, 59–72. doi:10.1080/17538150902779535.

Gudykunst, W. B., Gao, G., Schmidt, K. L., Nishida, T., Bond, M. H., Leung, K., & Barraclough, R. A. (1992). The influence of individualism-collectivism, self-monitoring, and predicted-outcome value on communication in ingroup and outgroup relationships. *Journal of Cross-Cultural Psychology, 23*, 196–213. doi:10.1177/0022022192232005

Hall, E. T. (1969). *The hidden dimension*. Garden City, NY: Doubleday.

Hofstede, G. (1980). *Culture's consequences*. Beverly Hills, CA: Sage.

Hsieh, Y. J. (2010). Cross-cultural communication: East vs. West. *Advances in International Marketing, 9*, 283. doi:10.1108/S14740-7979(2011)0000021015

Jain, S. L. (2013). *Malignant: How cancer becomes us*. Oakland, CA: University of California Press.

Jena, A. B., Olenski, A. R., & Blumenthal, D. M. (2016). Sex differences in physician salary in US public medical schools. *JAMA Internal Medicine*. doi:10.1001/jamainternmed.2016.3284

Johnson, S. K. (2002). Hmong health beliefs and experiences in the Western health care system. *Journal of Transcultural Nursing, 13*, 126–132.

Kakai, H. (2002). A double standard in bioethical reasoning for disclosure of advanced cancer diagnosis in Japan. *Health Communication, 14*, 361–376.

Kluckhohn, F. R., & Strodtbeck, F. (1961). *Variations in value orientations*. New York, NY: Row, Peterson.

Kreps, G. L., Neuhauser, L., Sparks, L., & Villagran, M. (2008). The power of community-based health communication interventions to promote cancer prevention and control for at-risk populations. *Patient Education and Counseling, 71*, 315–318.

Kreps, G. L., & Sparks, L. (2008). Meeting the health literacy needs of vulnerable populations. *Patient Education and Counseling, 71*, 328–332.

Long, S. O. (2000). Public passages, personal passages, and reluctant passages: Notes on investigating disclosure practices in Japan. *Journal of Medical Humanities, 21*, 3–13.

Malmusi, D., Artazcoz, L., Benach, J., & Borell, C. (2011). Perception of real illness? How chronic conditions contribute to gender inequities in self-rated health. *European Journal of Public Health*, *22*(6), 781–786.

Marin, G., & Marin, B. V. (1991). *Research with Hispanic populations*. Newbury Park, CA: Sage.

Marin, G., Marin, B. V., Perez-Stable, E. J., Sabogal, F., & Otero-Sabogal, R. (1990). Changes in information as a function of culturally appropriate smoking cessation community intervention for Hispanics. *American Journal of Community Psychology*, *18*, 847–864.

Marin, G., & Triandis, H. C. (1985). Allocentrism as an important characteristic of the behavior of Latin Americans and Hispanics. In R. Diaz-Guerrero (Ed.), *Cross-cultural and national studies in social psychology* (pp. 85–104). Amsterdam: Elsevier Science.

Meyer, E. (2014). *The culture map: Breaking through the invisible boundaries of global business*. New York, NY: Public Affairs.

Mok, E., & Martinson, I. (2000). Empowerment of Chinese patients with cancer through self-help groups in Hong Kong. *Cancer Nursing*, *23*, 206–213.

Mukherjee, S. (2010). *The emperor of all maladies*. New York, NY: Scribner.

Petronio, S. (2002). *Boundaries of privacy: Dialectics of disclosure*. Albany, NY: State University of New York Press.

Roberts, R. (2014). *Everybody's got something*. New York, NY: Grand Central.

Schwarz, N., Oyserman, D., & Peytcheva, E. (2010). Cognition, communication, and culture: Implications for the survey response process. In J. A. Harkness, M. Braun, B. Edwards, T. P. Johnson, L. Lyberg, P. P. Mohler, ..., T. W. Smith (Eds.), *Survey methods in multinational, multiregional, and multicultural contexts* (pp. 177–190). Hoboken, NJ: John Wiley & Sons. doi:10.1002/9780470609927.ch10

Sentell, T., Dela Cruz, M. R., Heo, H., & Braun, K. L. (2013). Health literacy, health communication challenges, and cancer screening among rural native Hawaiian and Filipino women. *Journal of Cancer Education*, *28*, 325–334. doi:10.1007/s13187-013-0471-3

Sentell, T. L., Tsoh, J. Y., Davis, T., Davis, J., & Braun, K. L. (2015). Low health literacy and cancer screening among Chinese Americans in California: A cross-sectional analysis. *BMJ Open*, *5*, e006104. doi:10.1136/bmjopen-2014-006104

Sherr, L. (2014). *Sally Ride: America's First Woman in Space*. New York, NY: Simon & Schuster.

Sparks, L. (2013). Health communication and caregiving research, policy, and practice. In R. C. Talley & S. S. Travis (Eds.), *Caregiving across the professions: A multi-disciplinary, coordinated perspective* (pp. 131–175). New York, NY: Springer.

Sparks, L., & Miller-Day, M. (2014). Methodological approaches to eliminating health disparities. In B. Whaley (Ed.), *Research methods in health communication: Principles and application* (pp. 318–336). New York, NY: Taylor and Francis.

Sparks, L., & Villagran, M. (2008). *La Comunicación en el Cancer: Comunicación y apoyo emocional en el laberinto del cancer*. [English translation: Communication and emotional support in the cancer maze.] Madrid, Spain: Aresta.

Sparks, L., & Villagran, M. (2010). *Patient and provider interaction: A global health communication perspective*. Cambridge: Polity Press.

Triandis, H. C., Marin, G., Hui, C. H., Lisansky, J., & Ottati, V. (1984). Role perceptions of Hispanic young adults. *Journal of Cross-Cultural Psychology*, *15*, 297–320.

World Health Organization. (2007). Unequal, unfair, ineffective and inefficient gender inequity in health. Report by the women and gender equity knowledge network. Geneva, Switzerland. Retrieved from http://www.who.int/social_determinants/resources/csdh_media/wgekn_final_report_07.pdf?ua=1

· 4 ·

WHO'S WHO

Social Identity and Cancer Care

Radiation and chemotherapy broke the ground.
She drank a glass of rainwater,

rousing the seeds.

When the incision was made, red petals bloomed
beneath the blade—

a clutch of tulips.

The surgeon plucked them out, pressing them
in a book for the tumor board.

—"Biopsy" by Stacy Nigliazzo

When Mary Lee was diagnosed with pancreatic cancer at the age of 71, she was running her own law practice. That work had shaped her life for many decades. Over the previous ten years, she'd cut back on the kinds and number of cases she accepted as she moved toward possible retirement, but she still had three employees and numerous clients. Even if treatment—starting with surgery—went well, she knew she would not be able to keep up with her clients' needs and court deadlines in the coming months. Though it was incredibly difficult for her to give up the work that she loved, she spent hours, in between doctor visits and medical tests, on the phone mapping out what needed to be done and making sure lawyers that she respected would take on specific clients and cases.

In some ways, these tasks invigorated Mary Lee and distracted her from thinking about her cancer. When she knew that all the details would be handled, she felt relieved not to worry about her clients' futures as she faced her own cancer treatment. She had done what she thought she needed do, and she took pride in seeing her work through. One day, when she called to talk with the administrative assistant who was helping wrap things up, she heard the automatic message stating that the office was permanently closed. She cried that day because she realized that she was no longer a practicing lawyer. Mary Lee's social identity was *attorney*, but cancer changed that part of how she thought about herself and approached her day-to-day life.

When Mary Lee was interviewed for an oral history project about her career years before her cancer diagnosis, the interviewer asked about her proudest accomplishment. Without taking time to think, she said that she was most proud of raising her two daughters. Because she had many professional accomplishments about which she had talked during the interview, her response about being a mother surprised her. Mary Lee's social identity was determined by her role in her family as well as her professional role in society.

Sometimes, we take for granted who we are, who others think we are, what we have accomplished, and how we, as individuals, contribute to others' lives. This chapter focuses on how individuals inhabit social identities, how others' perceptions influence our views of ourselves, and how cancer introduces a new identity for the patient and for the caregiver.

Whether you are a scholar of health communication or studying the field as a student or are a patient, a caregiver, or a healthcare provider, what would you say if asked to write a description of yourself based on what you value, the roles you play in others' lives, and who you consider yourself to be in the world? To answer this multifaceted question, you must consider your *social identity*. Social identity is the way we define ourselves and the way we are defined by others based on the formal and informal groups to which we belong.

Each of us belongs to several groups based on the roles we play, and those groups shape our identities. We each carry labels that others see. Mary Lee, for instance, carried labels like *mother*, *lawyer*, *world traveler*, and *Cubs fan*. Those who knew her as a lawyer may not have thought of her as a baseball fan. Not all aspects of a person's social identity are visible to everyone with whom that person interacts.

Who Are You? The Authors Reveal Their Social Identities

While this book is about patients, caregivers, and healthcare providers, the authors want to take this opportunity to share our own social identities as examples of how two individuals with some social roles in common answer that multifaceted question differently. Both authors are White, female, and in our early fifties. We are both well educated, having each earned a Ph.D., and we have chosen to work as professors at the same university. But we have different social identities, different ways we define ourselves, and different ways others perceive us.

Lisa Sparks:

> I am a scholar–teacher of health and cancer communication science and a university professor and the dean of the School of Communication at Chapman University. I truly enjoy serving the students and having the opportunity to help and work with our amazing and dedicated faculty to build the School of Communication into one of the best in the nation. I love to write and consider myself to be a creative thinker and a person who can generate interesting ideas into action. I am a mom of three adorable girls (Elena, Arianna, and Athena) who are incredibly special to me yet also drive me crazy at times as I try to raise them to be independent young women of character. I am a devoted and loving wife and dedicated parent. I am an avid runner and rather sporty girl but always need more time to train. I love to play (and watch) tennis, but am now prone to injuries and so cannot play to the level I did when I was a teenager, which can be really frustrating! I also love to go hiking and skiing and travel to interesting places with my family, as these activities create wonderful family stories, experiences, and memories. I am not a morning person. I am a coffee fanatic. I am a bit of a Francophile but married to an Italian who loves me despite that. I am an art lover with a background in art history and photography and a general lover of the arts including live theatre performances, musical theatre, and opera. I am a pseudo-connoisseur of California chardonnay and, through the influence of my Italian spouse over the years, I have grown to love and appreciate the robust Italian reds such as Barolo, Barbaresco, Sangiovese, and varied Chianti wines. I am an Episcopalian (Christian) but enjoy Buddhist philosophy, readings, and meditation. I am a Western girl who loves classical music and all sorts of alternative music but who has grown to also love country music. Although I am a health nut most of the time, I truly enjoy food including a fabulous burger, steak, or barbeque. Finally, I will always consider myself to be a caregiver. First, to my dad who

> died of lung cancer in 1997. Although I had been studying issues surrounding health communication and aging since 1992, it was after this experience that I devoted my life's work to the study of cancer communication science. More recently, I am also increasingly taking on additional care for my aging mom as well. We moved her from Oklahoma to Orange County several years ago so we can keep a closer eye on her as she enters her golden years! P.S. She loves the sunny OC life!

Lisa lists her current work first, perhaps because authors and academics grow used to doing that in biographical notes publishers require. Certainly, the most prominent aspect of social identity that the two of us have in relation to this project are *author* and *professor*. Lisa's description of herself also reveals her role as mother and wife, her interests and leisure activities, and her personality traits.

If Anna Leahy were to compare herself directly to Lisa, she might reveal that she prefers red wine to white and, though she exercises sometimes, would not call herself *avid* and would not call what she does *training*. In fact, she does not mention her own physicality or spirituality (she was raised Catholic and went to Catholic schools from kindergarten through high school) in her self-description.

Anna Leahy:

> I'm a writer—poetry, nonfiction, and, occasionally, fiction. By the time I was four years old, I hoarded paper and scrawled on a yellow legal pad next to my mother's desk as she wrote there. I'm also a university professor and, more recently, the director for undergraduate research and creative activity, which demands more multitasking and is rewarding because I can see the end results of my efforts in what students are able to accomplish. In college, I rarely spoke in class, and teaching was one of the last things I thought I would ever do. Teaching assistantships were a way for me to go to graduate school to practice creative writing under the guidance of mentors. I enjoy hanging out with writers and other professors and talking about big ideas and minutia. Realizing that I had become a better teacher over years of practice, I started to study pedagogy more consciously and now write about teaching, too. I'm a curious person, interested in a wide array of subjects, a characteristic my father especially encouraged in me. I co-wrote a book with my husband about the end of the space shuttle program. We are both interested in aviation, spaceflight, and science, and we enjoy writing, reading, and travel. Our trips to Florida for the last space shuttles launches were among the best experiences of our lives, and we've been to France twice in the last couple of years. I think of myself as a good collaborator because I'm relatively patient, straightforward, and detail oriented, especially in editing. Writing with someone else requires the right mix of skills, expertise, and personality in the other person, too. Mary Lee and Andy in this book are my parents. Both died of cancer, and that's why I wanted to be part of this book project and also wrote another book called *Tumor*.

While Anna's writing often reveals personal information and family relationships, her description here focuses more on her public social identities and how she wants to be perceived by readers of this book. She refers to her past personal experiences as having shaped her present professional self.

These are the authors' current identities. Social identities shift over time and as our lives change. While Anna may still listen to the 80s music she first heard in college (and is surprised that her students thirty years later know those songs), she does not behave in exactly the same ways she did then. Importantly, given the focus of *Conversing with Cancer,* both authors have parents who have had cancer. That experience changed how we think of ourselves. We have a personal stake in this book. The authors of this book have not faced that diagnosis themselves, however. Not yet, though statistics indicate that there is a chance one of us will be diagnosed with cancer someday.

The labels a person wears are determined, in part, by how that person understands oneself and what that person projects to others, which varies according to the social circumstances. Different people may know us in different ways. One paragraph does not capture all a person's social identities. People also sometimes wear labels that others assign to them, whether they think of themselves that way or not.

Social Identity Theory: The Basics

Some labels are chosen and cultivated, and others emerge out of life's happenstance. Health communication experts see these issues—identities, labels, and their effects—as part of *Social Identity Theory* (SIT) and have used SIT to understand communication issues surrounding cancer diagnosis, treatment, recovery, and end-of-life. SIT is a broad theory of group relations that focuses on the meaning people assign to their identities, the ways in which they guard those identities and meanings, and the ways in which they respond when identities are in jeopardy. SIT deals primarily with identification within large social groups such as age, gender, or culture, and you may be familiar with some of these ideas from our discussion of culture and cancer in Chapter 3.

SIT can also be applied to smaller and more specialized groups such as a family unit, a professional affiliation, or a group with a specific disease, such as cancer. Cancer is statistically linked with certain societal groups, including older adults, smokers, and excessive sunbathers. For any cancer patient, no matter what the person's group affiliations or identity labels, it is important to look at how our identities shape our attitudes and how we behave.

Strongly identifying with a particular group that engages in certain preventative practices increases the likelihood that the individual will practice appropriate cancer prevention strategies (Harwood & Sparks, 2003; Sparks & Harwood, 2008). Women who strongly view themselves as women—who see that label as an important part of their social identity—may be more likely to get regular Pap smears and mammograms or do breast self-exams regularly. On the other hand, if a person does not strongly identify with a particular group membership, that person is less likely to enact practices common for that group. If someone smokes two packs of cigarettes a day but does not think of oneself as a heavy smoker, that person might not worry about lung cancer.

The body is the first casualty of the happenstance of cancer, but social identity often suffers too. Throughout our lives, certain aspects of who we are become more or less important. Being a cancer patient is not a welcome identity but does become important for the person diagnosed with cancer. As S. Lochlann Jain (2013) wrote in her book *Malignant*, "I didn't know the least thing about my new role. I could more or less enact curiosity-driven researcher, loving girlfriend, stern teacher, doting Mima, dependable big sister, cash-strapped daughter, fun-loving chum, polite dinner guest, competent student, active teammate…but sick patient? Not in my repertoire" (p. 3).

Communication is the means by which a cancer patient and also caregivers and healthcare providers help create meaning for the experience and shape the patient's transformed identity. Awareness of social identity can help cancer patients, caregivers, and providers be more active participants in fostering a positive social identity.

When an individual is diagnosed with cancer, it is easy for that individual—and those around that person—to let go of the social identity that existed prior to diagnosis. A person who was viewed as *a friend* becomes *a friend with cancer*, or *an athlete* becomes *a former athlete* because of cancer. Someone might whisper as a woman in a wig passes, *Do you think she has cancer?* When undergoing chemotherapy treatment, baldness, weight loss (or weight gain from steroids), or a portable chemo pump may mark a patient physically so that even strangers think: *person with cancer*. Cancer-related identity transformation is common after diagnosis and during treatment, and an individual's social identity can be eclipsed by the presence of illness. Past accomplishments and current roles seem to fade or be overshadowed with that label: *person with cancer*. As one's previous identity transforms, it can seem as if those qualities that established likeness with others or that distinguished one in particular ways are obscured by the fact of cancer. Family, friends, or coworkers may want to talk about the person with cancer outside of that individual's presence or avoid talking about cancer when the individual is present.

The tendency by others to make note of this fact of cancer is often intended in a positive way, perhaps to alert people to be extra-kind about physical signs of illness or to be especially understanding when the person misses a meeting or has specific scheduling requests. Miriam Engelberg (2006), in her biting memoir-in-comics, pokes fun at her new label of *person with cancer*. In a strip called "Diagnosis," she tries to restrain her tell-all tendencies but ends up announcing her new label—*I have breast cancer*—to everyone she encounters. To inform colleagues of her diagnosis without a series of emotional interactions, she sends an email about a new Excel manual but uses *I have breast cancer* in the subject line of the message. Later, when she gets bad news from her physician, she writes to her boss to say she will stop in to pick up a few things but does not want to talk about her cancer; when she arrives at the office, people come up with excuses to flee. Through exaggeration, Engelberg shows how people interacted with her differently because she became part of a new group and had a new social identity: *person with cancer*. She also points out that she sometimes acted in ways that surprised her.

Some cancer patients appreciate the new attention and generosity. Patricia Grace King (2014) donned a bright pink wig when she faced baldness as a side effect of chemotherapy treatment for her breast cancer and wore it to teach her creative writing class; she liked the attention, found that the wig deflected her baldness, and wanted to portray strength. Engelberg (2006) used her diagnosis to silence telemarketers, inserting the information into conversations with strangers so that conversation was halted. Other patients, though, bristle at the new attention, in part because they consider illness a private matter. Still others feel as if nothing the cancer patient has ever done—or will ever do—matters because the only thing on everyone's mind is cancer. This perception of one's own social identity can lead to feeling stereotyped and to feelings of hopelessness or isolation. For many cancer patients, whether they appreciate attention or not, the way the world views who they are is no longer firmly rooted in a set of group affiliations formed over time. Instead, identity is now formed or influenced by membership in one group: people who have been diagnosed with cancer.

Whether you are a patient, a caregiver, or a healthcare provider, you may want to consider your social identity and think about how it influences your day-to-day actions, thoughts, and feelings as well as your larger goals. The following may help a person think about who you are in the world and about how others perceive you:

- How long have you lived where you live now—the house, the town? Do you like your home and your neighborhood? Have you moved around during your life? If so, how did each place influence your life differently?
- Do you have a job or career? If so, do you enjoy that work? Have your ideas about your job(s) changed over time?
- Are you single, married, or in an intimate relationship? If so, how would you describe that relationship and what it contributes to your life?
- Do you have children? Do you have parents? If so, do they live in the same home with you, nearby, or far away?
- Do you value time alone? If so, what kinds of things do you do when you are by yourself?
- Do you value informal social time with others? Do you enjoy spending time with longtime friends? Do you enjoy meeting new people?
- Do you belong to any organizations, perhaps a church, a book club, or a gym? If so, how do those activities and interacting with the people there contribute to your life?
- Do you enjoy listening to music, reading books, watching television, participating in sports, traveling, gardening, or knitting? What hobbies or pastimes interest you?
- Do you know others with cancer—or who are caregivers or healthcare providers? How does being part of this group influence your life?
- Write one paragraph describing yourself, as this book's authors did at the beginning of this chapter. What does that summary reveal?

An Astronaut Gets Cancer: How Social Identity Shapes Care

Sally Ride, the first American woman in space, seemed to be more aware of her social identity than most of us. She had strived for decades to keep her personal life out of public view. When she was diagnosed with pancreatic cancer, she worried about how her identity would be transformed. For one thing, having cancer did not sync up with how she thought of herself or how she wanted others to think of her. As her biographer Lynn Sherr (2014) wrote, "How could Sally, a fitness fanatic who, at fifty-nine, was in better shape than most teenagers, have cancer?" The label *fitness fanatic* was part of her social identity, and she did not want others to label her as *person with cancer* instead.

Ride was also concerned that this new label would affect her work at Sally Ride Science, her positions on various boards, and the way people viewed her former employer, NASA. She would never have worn a pink wig to board meetings, as Patricia did to class. At first, only her healthcare providers and Tam O'Shaughnessy, her life partner, knew about the diagnosis. When she and O'Shaughnessy told some managers at Sally Ride Science about the illness, they did not reveal that the diagnosis was cancer. It was a few months before Ride told her sister. Ride went through a six-hour surgery; lost weight, dropping to a hundred pounds; and wore a natural-looking wig after she lost her hair during chemotherapy. As Sherr (2014) wrote about the year following the diagnosis, "Sally's random bursts of energy, combined with her perennial upbeat outlook, likely convinced her that she would make it, that she could be one of the few who beat the odds. It certainly kept her illness off the public radar" (p. 309). Ride thought she would make it and, therefore, probably did not want others to doubt that future or re-label her.

Energy, endurance, and optimism were part of Ride's personality and also qualities related to her social identities as astronaut, scientist, and advocate for girls' education. As Sherr (2014) put it, when she made the decision to move forward with treatment, "Sally moved into mission mode. The engineer in her saw a problem to be solved; the scientist, an unknown to be explored. She got out her notebook and made a new set of checklists" (p. 303). She researched nutrition and cancer, then started a vegan diet. She researched attitudes and cancer, then stopped watching television news full of negative stories and, just as we suggest in this book, focused on positive thoughts and conversations. She continued to exercise and added meditation and acupuncture. She clung to her social identity and used the ways she thought about herself to face her cancer diagnosis and treatment with action.

Ride was, in fact, such a logical thinker—someone who trained for all possibilities and tackled problems head on—that she and O'Shaughnessy planned Ride's memorial service together. "They picked the site, the speakers, the tulips and the open bar." Sherr describes this planning session, with Ride in the hospital bed in her bedroom because she was too weak to walk downstairs, as "a welcome respite from their grief" (p. 311). Ride's social identity—the roles she held, the ways she thought of herself and others thought of her—shaped her attitudes toward cancer and how she behaved as a cancer patient. She likely wanted to ensure that she would be remembered by those social identities she had cultivated before she had cancer. And after years of keeping her relationship with O'Shaugnessy a secret, she gave her partner the okay to reveal their domestic partnership after she had died, thereby accepting publicly a social identity with which she had lived privately for decades.

On July 23, 2012, sixteen months after the cancer diagnosis, Sally Ride died. And shortly thereafter, the world, including many of her friends, found out for the first time that she had been a *person with cancer*. Few individuals guard—are able to guard or even want to guard—their social identities as vigilantly as Ride did hers. Her desire for privacy while being a public figure demonstrate the range of issues involved when an individual's social identity is transformed by cancer.

It is important to keep in mind that different people handle a cancer diagnosis and sharing information differently. Television host Robin Roberts (2014), in her book *Everybody's Got Something*, provides a good reminder to all of us not to judge others. Like Sally Ride, writer Nora Ephron did not share her diagnosis widely. Of that decision, Roberts writes, "What I know is this: Each of our journeys is different and personal. There's not a one-size-fits-all when it comes to this or any other type of life-threatening illness or challenge. You've got to do what is best for you" (p. 82). Each patient must decide for oneself when, how, and with whom to share information about a cancer diagnosis and treatment.

Social Identity and Caregivers

Sally Ride's primary caregiver and life partner, Tam O'Shaughnessy, guarded their social identities as well. She confided the news with a few people close to her, possibly, at least in part, because she needed emotional support as a caregiver. Cancer not only has the ability to redefine the way others view the social identity of a cancer patient but also can affect family members and caregivers of the patient. Even when the patient and the caregiver are not perceived by those labels by others, they still inhabit those roles in their day-to-day lives. Priorities and interests may shift. Some patients and caregivers, like Ride and O'Shaughnessy, remove themselves from social and work obligations—narrow their previous social identities—so that they can concentrate on the treatment phase of the cancer continuum. After successful treatment for breast cancer, musician Melissa Etheridge and actor Christina Applegate became health activists, using their cancer experiences in their public lives. The cancer diagnosis, treatment schedule, side effects of treatment, and progression of the disease affect the decisions, schedules, and interactions of the patient and the caregiver.

As we discuss at greater length in Chapter 8, the role of caregiver can be emotionally taxing, physically demanding, and time-consuming. Because of these wide-ranging demands, caregivers' social identities are often transformed by their involvement in the continuum of cancer care. When Lisa Sparks, one of this book's authors, was caring for her father as he was dying of lung cancer, the caregiver role became a dominant aspect of her identity, both in the way others viewed her and in her view of herself. During that time, caregiving tasks shaped her daily schedule and longer-term plans, and the challenges and joys associated with caregiving became frequent topics of conversation. Now, nearly two decades later, the past experience of being a caregiver remains a part of her identity, but that label does not have the prominence it did when she was living that role every day. Looking more closely at social identity theory, with both patient and caregiver in mind, can help scholars, students, and those directly involved in the continuum of cancer care understand how our identities—our views and others' views based on our roles in the world—evolve during cancer care.

Who's Your Tribe?

SIT—social identity theory—includes the notion that our identities are shaped by our relationship and interaction with groups, which can be categorized as primary, secondary, and tertiary identities or groups. Different researchers use these categories in different ways to look at and categorize social groups (e.g., Harwood & Sparks, 2003).

In one useful way to look at the role of groups in social identity formation, primary groups are those cultural groups like the ones we discussed in Chapter 3, groups based on age, gender, ethnicity, and so on. While some researchers define primary categories differently, it is helpful to think of primary groups as those a person does not choose, whereas secondary groups are more fluid social groups that a person chooses. People come and go from such secondary groups based on needs and interests. The workplace, in which membership involves the exchange of money, is an example of a secondary group.

When applied to health or cancer communication, groups associated with health behaviors can be considered secondary groups. Examples of secondary groups include smokers, couch potatoes, runners, and gym nuts. A person who thinks of oneself as a smoker, for instance, may have a more difficult time quitting the habit than someone who smokes but does not think of oneself as a smoker. A person who lives near the beach or sees oneself as tan may struggle to change behaviors to reduce the risk of skin cancer.

But where does *person with cancer* fit into group identity? It is not an inherent trait like gender or age. But it is not a group anyone would choose either.

A third level of social identity—what the authors of *Conversing with Cancer* think of as *tertiary groups*—is associated with cancer. For the new patient, this tertiary group feels neither long-term nor close-knit, though, over time, many cancer patients feel camaraderie or a bond with other cancer patients.

The cancer patient, the caregiver, and others may also think more specifically in terms like *cancer victim* and *cancer survivor*. Thinking of oneself as a victim may lead to the lessening of guilt, which can be a relief. Or it can lead to behavior that undermines decision-making, action, and treatment results because one feels helpless. Thinking of oneself as a survivor can foster a social identity that conveys strength and looking forward. Tertiary social identity, then, affects one's psychological orientation toward one's circumstances and, ultimately, one's behavior and interactions (e.g., Harwood & Sparks, 2003). Common ways people view and talk about cancer are discussed more extensively in Chapter 9. The point in relation to social identity is that membership in this tertiary group—people with cancer—comes with some built-in cultural attitudes and language that group members tend to understand and, to different extents, use.

There exists no right or wrong way to view cancer, of course. In addition, your attitude as a patient or caregiver may shift day to day or over time. Some days, you may feel as if cancer is a battleground. Other days, you may feel as if you are in the midst of a transformative journey. Sometimes, anger—and the energy that comes with it—may be helpful. At other times, anger may undermine your progress. You may feel increased awareness of your priorities, or you may feel as if enlightenment falsely glamorizes your illness. No matter the patient's attitude, understanding one's tertiary identity—the patient's relationship to cancer—can help that person negotiate decisions and behaviors related to cancer care.

Cancer Stereotypes and Discrimination: Impediments to Care

Belonging to a group, of course, brings with it the risk of *discrimination*, or judgment based on that group membership or label rather than based on the individual. Not surprisingly, research reveals that discrimination as a result of group membership can cause stress (Harwood & Sparks, 2003; Sparks & Harwood, 2008; Villagran & Sparks, 2010). A cancer diagnosis creates a stressful situation, and bias against cancer patients from others can compound that stress. SIT provides an explanation for the origins of stereotypes and discriminatory behaviors. Understanding the origins of stereotypes and discriminatory behaviors can help a cancer patient or caregiver negotiate communication and decision-making that is related to cancer care (Harwood & Sparks, 2003).

If a person is a member of a particular group, that individual may be judged to possess all of the characteristics socially attributed to that group. That is not fair, but it happens a lot. A physician or caregiver, for example, may assume that someone with gray hair who looks frail is confused because she is elderly rather than because she is dehydrated. A caregiver may not pay enough attention to advancing neuropathy in the feet of a patient who already walked with a cane before the diagnosis. A healthcare provider may assume that the Chinese woman undergoing treatment is a healthy eater with a diet of mostly fish, rice, and vegetables, though she might eat most of her meals at a fast-food chain near her home. These are mistakes made when someone stereotypes, or applies all socially constructed characteristics of a social group to an individual person, instead of recognizing that individual group members vary widely.

In other words, identities including stereotypes of and assumptions about social groups can influence diagnosis and treatment in subtle and important ways (Harwood & Sparks, 2003; Sparks & Harwood, 2008). Physicians may stereotype their patients and, often unintentionally, use stereotypes in the diagnosis or treatment of medical complaints. When this occurs, physicians tend to perceive complaints as aligned with commonly known risk factors for the identity groups to which the patient is known to belong. For example, younger patients' symptoms may be overlooked because they are at lower risk for cancer, which may prevent them from receiving diagnostic tests that would be routine in older patients. Or older adults' symptoms might be perceived as a normal part of aging, which may prevent them from receiving alleviation of treatment side effects that would be routine in younger patients. That is not fair. That is detrimental to a patient's health and well-being. Stereotypes can interfere with the goal for the cancer patient to live the best life possible.

Patients, caregivers, and healthcare providers who are aware of SIT can use the ideas presented here to recognize and avoid stereotyping and discriminatory behavior as well as to understand the importance of group membership in shaping social identity.

Social Identity and Cancer Care

Every person has a social identity. A greater understanding of how social identity functions in the continuum of cancer care can help create practical strategies that are theoretically based to guide patients and providers as they create, re-create, negotiate, and renegotiate their own and each other's identities across the *continuum of cancer care*, which encompasses prevention, detection, diagnosis, treatment, survivorship, and end-of-life. When patients, caregivers, and providers keep their own and each other's social identities in mind, they can communicate more effectively and make more appropriate decisions. Only by understanding the balance between belonging to social groups and having individual traits can the patient and provider work toward the best possible care and the best decision-making in that patient's situation.

The next chapter extends some of the ideas about social identity from this chapter. In particular, Chapter 5 focuses on the role that patient age plays in cancer care. As discussed at the beginning of Chapter 4, age is a primary social group, one we do not choose. As we move from one stage of life to another, we move from one age-based social group to another. As we shift from childhood to adulthood and then from middle age to senior citizen, our priorities, attitudes, and approaches tend to shift. Whether the patient is a child, in middle age, or elderly affects how the patient, family, caregiver, and provider negotiate a diagnosis and treatment. That is why age is one aspect of social identity that deserves an entire chapter.

Exercise & Discussion

Task

1) Each student should think of two aspects of their identity that are crucial. Consider the strongest in-group affiliations you have. Consider

whether you identify most strongly with your work, your family, your leisure activities, or an aspect of cultural identity discussed in Chapter 3.

2) Consider what would happen if one of those aspects of your identity were stripped away from you. Consider how you would feel if both aspects of your identity were stripped away.

Sharing

Discuss the above self-awareness task and how it might relate to a cancer diagnosis. Who are we without our identity? What makes us the people that we are, and how do we cope when part of our identity is no longer a part of us? How do we feel and cope when we are no longer in a role with which we strongly identify or no longer feel needed in that role? How can we hold onto aspects of identity when life circumstances change? What means can we use to create a new identity when our old one does not work? Discuss how these questions relate to the identity and daily life of a cancer patient.

References

Engelberg, M. (2006). *Cancer made me a shallower person: A memoir in comics*. New York, NY: Harper.

Harwood, J., & Sparks, L. (2003). Social identity and health: An intergroup communication approach to cancer. *Health Communication*, *15*, 145–170.

Jain, S. L. (2013). *Malignant: How cancer becomes us*. Oakland, CA: University of California Press.

King, P. G. (2014). Personal Blog. Retrieved from http://www.patriciagraceking.com/blog

Roberts, R. (2014) *Everybody's got something*. New York, NY: Grand Central.

Sherr, L. (2014). *Sally ride: America's first woman in space*. New York, NY: Simon & Schuster.

Sparks, L., & Harwood, J. (2008). Cancer, aging, and social identity: Development of an integrated model of social identity theory and health communication. In L. Sparks, H. D. O'Hair, & G. L. Kreps (Eds.), *Cancer communication and aging* (pp. 77–95). Cresskill, NJ: Hampton Press.

Villagran, M. M., & Sparks, L. (2010). Social identity and health contexts. In H. Giles, S. A. Reid, & J. Harwood (Eds.), *The dynamics of intergroup communication* (pp. 235–248). New York, NY: Peter Lang.

· 5 ·

CITIZENS OF CANCER LAND

Cancer Communication Across a Lifetime

Now she allows certain words to enter her body.
Peering at jaundiced skin in the mirror and cola-colored
pee in the toilet, she sees how ignorant we are
of our inner lives, the continual beating of ventricles,
the exchange of oxygen and carbon dioxide in alveoli.

She thinks, *I've never seen the size or shape of my liver.*

Cancer speaks in covert tongues, like toddlers with magic
words: *Kalibushti!* or *Slagermosh!* But we are exoskeletons,
vain and lordly, thinking we are hair, skin, nails, teeth, smile.
She tries to say certain words to her husband, her daughter,
but cancer speaks for itself. Towards the end, she stops
speaking in native voice, begins to speak only in god-tongue.

—"Exoskeleton" by Risa Denenberg

Lucy Grealy was nine years old when a playground accident led to the discovery that she had Ewing's sarcoma, which then led to years of treatment that involved surgery, chemotherapy, and radiation. Even as an adult, she underwent reconstructive surgery numerous times as a result of her earlier cancer. She also continued to grapple emotionally with the effects of having had cancer that altered her appearance and shaped her approach to life.

Because she was very young when she was diagnosed and treated for cancer, Lucy Grealy's doctors, nurses, and parents did not share with her all the details of her situation, and she was not always able to make full sense of what she heard and felt. Grealy (2003) wrote, "Every day I'd have some test, and it never occurred to me to ask what was going on, what the tests were for, what the results were. At least this is how I remember it, though my mother tells it differently" (p. 42). The patient and the patient's family have different experiences of the cancer care continuum. In this case, the patient and her mother remember the experience differently, in part because the patient was a child when she was diagnosed with and treated for cancer.

As an adult writing about her experience with cancer, Grealy (2003) remembers, "There were definite problems to face here, but to me they seemed entirely manageable: lie still when you're told, be brave. It didn't seem so much to ask, really, considering what I got in return: attention, absence from school, occasional presents, and, though I wouldn't have admitted it to anyone even if I could have articulated it, freedom from tensions at home" (p. 38). In fact, it was only years later that she really understood that she'd had cancer.

Lucy's experience as a cancer patient was shaped by her age and her childhood outlook on life. A man in his forties, perhaps with a family, a job, and a monthly mortgage or rent payment, would have a very different experience as a cancer patient. And a woman diagnosed, say, with breast cancer in her eighties would have a very different experience as a patient than that man in his forties. This chapter takes into account the role that stage of life plays for the cancer patient and family and also what kinds of information—including prevention—we need at which stages of our lives.

Talking with Children About Cancer

Children with Cancer

Serious illness or death of a child is something that parents hope will never happen in their family. Cancer in a child is indeed rare, so most families never face a situation in which a child is diagnosed with cancer. Yet, according to the National Cancer Institute, "cancer is the leading cause of disease-related death among children and adolescents." Survival rates for childhood cancer are generally good, with more than 80% of patients living at least five years. The most common type of childhood cancer is acute lymphoblastic leukemia, and children with Down Syndrome are at slightly higher risk for this cancer. Its five-year survival rate has improved from less than 10% in the 1960s to a very encouraging 90% in this century (NCI, 2016). While prognosis varies by cancer type and stage, the outlook for the child is often good. Each diagnosis and patient is a distinct, individual situation, and children deal with illness and stress differently than adults.

When a child is diagnosed with cancer, the communication process and modes can be very different than when an adult is diagnosed with cancer. The first major difference is that, in the United States, the physician typically discusses the diagnosis with the patient's parents or legal guardians before informing the patient. Depending on the age of the child, healthcare providers may discuss the diagnosis with the parents in very different words and scope than they discuss the situation with the child. In other words, because of age, the patient may be given limited information and develop limited understanding of the situation (Harzold & Sparks, 2007).

Research indicates that, particularly in cases of pediatric cancer, parents establish the initial privacy rules that define how to regulate information about the illness and navigate the difficult conversation path along the family's journey through cancer (Bylund, Galvin, Dunet, & Reyes, 2011; Harzold & Sparks, 2007). This aspect of ongoing communication emerges from the initial communication process established when the cancer is diagnosed. In most cases, the child should be told at least generally about the illness, given some terminology, and told some of what to expect so that the child has ways of talking about the situation, sets appropriate expectations, and can communicate about symptoms and side effects. But that may be impossible with very young children. Some children who are old enough to understand their situations may be involved in decision-making about their own health care, but, ultimately, parents or legal guardians will usually make decisions about treatment of their children.

As treatment moves forward, children may experience side effects, which can be physically and emotionally painful and which may be observable to others, including other children. These experiences make open communication important so that the child has some understanding of what is truly happening to one's own body and some understanding of others' reactions.

According to researchers Michael K. Cruce and Terry Stinnet (2006), children with cancer are more likely to face problems at school. Children with cancer may be more socially withdrawn, and their peers may not understand serious illness. In addition, as a result of some cancer treatments, pediatric patients may exhibit cognitive side effects, like what adults call chemo brain. Because of physical, psychological, and emotional changes resulting from the disease and treatment, pediatric cancer patients may struggle academically even if they had excelled academically before diagnosis and are physically responding well to treatment. Children may miss school for doctor appointments and treatments as well as when they are not feeling well. Parents and teachers must work together to ensure the patient can be as successful as possible in school and to encourage positive interactions between the patient and classmates.

A child with cancer may be absent from school for long periods of time or for short periods frequently. These interruptions and returns can be difficult to manage academically, emotionally, and socially. Cruce and Stinnet (2006) point to distraction, absenteeism, and refusal to do schoolwork as common issues for students who have cancer. To address the sometimes difficult transition between cancer treatment and school, some large healthcare organizations offer programs designed to help parents and teachers reintegrate children into school. Such programs educate the adults involved in a child's school life and also give them the language and practical skills to address the situation. A psychologist may also help prepare the child to return to the classroom, and Cruce and Stinnet (2006) suggest that pediatric cancer patients who perceive high support from classmates exhibit lower levels of avoidance behavior. Again, adults must work together and establish useful communication in order to foster an educational environment in which the patient can thrive.

Cruce and Stinnet (2006) also point out that children with cancer are not routinely screened for psychological conditions like depression or anxiety, even though they may exhibit symptoms. The healthcare team sees treating cancer as the priority and focuses on that biomedical problem. A diagnosis and medical treatment can make a child afraid. Symptoms like loss of energy or loss of appetite that might be diagnosed as depression in a healthy child may be side effects of the cancer treatment. If adults report experiencing chemo brain, for instance, there is no reason to think that children do not experience that side effect even if they do not understand the colloquial term for or good ways to describe cognitive symptoms.

Looking back on their experiences with childhood cancer, adult survivors and their parents recommend the following three approaches for families: 1) take one day at a time, 2) talk openly about the cancer, and 3) emphasize the normal aspects of living (Galvin et al., 2012; also see Harold & Sparks, 2007). These approaches benefit not only the patient but also the parents, who bear tremendous stress in these situations, as well as other family members, friends, and even the child's classmates.

Adulthood After Childhood Cancer

Adult survivors of childhood cancer may continue to experience their lives as shaped, at least in part, by their earlier illness. They may need lifelong follow-up care or health monitoring beyond what is usually recommended for adults in good health or may carry visible or physical signs of their earlier illness, such as an amputated limb. They may be more susceptible to chronic disease, suffer long-term side effects or long-term health risks from cancer treatment, and face psychological difficulties such as uncertainty about the future (Robinson & Hudson, 2014). Parents, too, may experience worry and strain for years, even after the child is an adult. Regardless of long-term consequences, ongoing, honest communication can help adult survivors of childhood cancer and their families cope over a lifetime and build healthy, happy lives.

As *Pilgrim Steps* blogger Jana Remy (2013) writes of her experiences with childhood bone cancer, "Even though thirty years have now passed since I first heard that dreadful cancer word spoken in connection with the symptoms of my own body, I still find it difficult to comprehend the life-changing event that was my diagnosis and treatment for osteosarcoma." The memory of the childhood cancer experience can make it seem distant or even as if it happened to a different person. "As I look back on what I went through then," Remy says, "it remains a kind of encapsulated moment that is hard for me to connect with now." The adult may see the relationship between illness and treatment differently than the child. In fact, anyone who survives cancer may develop a more positive outlook on what was an extraordinarily difficult period of life. "But what I remember most significantly was the feeling that the temporary horror of my cancer treatments was worthwhile to endure because of the possibility of eradicating my disease, and I trusted that my doctors were giving me the treatments that would increase my odds for survival."

As an adult looking back, Remy (2013) wonders whether her trust of the healthcare system and the physicians within it was naïve and whether, had she been older and able to make her own decisions, she would have agreed to surgery and chemotherapy. She understands that, especially because she was young, her culture—her family, her larger community in Utah—shaped what happened to her. And what happened to her continues to shape her life, as Remy (2008) walks through life on "a prosthetic leg with a computer-controlled knee joint" at a cost of more than $50,000. "Of course," Remy (2013) says, "with 30 years of hindsight it seems to have been a wise choice."

Perhaps that is the most important point to keep in mind when considering childhood cancer and a child's long-term survival. The goal is for that child to have decades of hindsight, even though children do not yet have the life experiences and perspective to view a cancer diagnosis, decisions, and treatment with the same long view as adults.

Children Who Have Loved Ones with Cancer

Sometimes a parent is the person with cancer; sometimes it is a grandparent or family friend. Regardless of who has cancer, there are several ways to help children feel safe and secure after the cancer diagnosis of a loved one. Communicating with children about a family member's or friend's cancer diagnosis can be a very emotional conversation, especially for the adult. These conversations, however, can also be opportunities for children to learn about the body, cancer, the power of medicine, and adults' love for them. The most important thing in a cancer conversation, as with any conversation with a child, is to convey that the child is and will be loved.

As Harzold and Sparks (2007) point out, the first step in communicating with children about cancer is to consider the audience. One must consider the child in terms of biological age, level of emotional growth, and intellectual ability to comprehend the situation, including the biomedical reality. Chronological age is often used as a predictor of how a child will react to being told someone has cancer, but the developmental and emotional maturity of the individual child is also a key consideration before beginning a discussion about cancer. When conversing with younger children about emotionally or intellectually challenging topics, props such as stuffed animals or books can be helpful in fostering more open, clear communication. Older children may have—or may appear to have—a clearer understanding of the meaning of cancer, but an adult should not assume that any individual fully understands such a complex disease or its effects. Children tend to take what you say literally and also pay attention to your tone of voice. Children need specific but personalized information to help them understand the cancer situation, the cancer care continuum, and their role in it.

Let's say that you are a parent who wants to talk to your child about your own parent's cancer diagnosis and upcoming treatment. As you analyze the audience by assessing your child, you should also think about key ideas, main points, and also the best words and phrases to use to describe the cancer situation. What is the most important information you want to convey? What are the simplest terms you can use to convey that information? Someone nervous about having a difficult conversation may build confidence by rehearsing the initial statements—aloud or silently—before speaking with the child. There is no need for a script or to memorize the whole conversation ahead of time. Like most spontaneous conversations, it should evolve naturally and allow for the child to determine what is covered. The most comfortable approach for both adult and child is often to allow information dissemination, questions by each participant, and answers to occur spontaneously, even if you have factual information you want to be sure to convey.

As you talk with a child, you probably want to frame the situation in a positive light, and you may be tempted to lie in hopes of allaying the child's fears. Lying, however, can be very detrimental to children and can lead to hurt feelings, especially if they later find out from someone else that what you told them is not true. Also, one should be cognizant of word choice. For instance, a child who hears that cancer is like a monster who needs to be blasted away may think that an actual monster lives inside a loved one's body. In these conversations, one should strive to be positive, but also be honest and realistic.

When Mary Lee Leahy told her daughters, Anna (one of this book's authors) and Brigid, that their father, who was 48 years old, had cancer, she was clear and honest but did not share many details in that initial conversation. Mary Lee was still grappling with the news herself, and her daughters were only 15 and 13 years old. She made it clear that their father's illness was very serious, but she did not share the then-terrible prognosis that he was likely to live for just a few weeks. She explained that he would start chemotherapy in a couple of days, so the girls knew what was going to happen in the immediate future.

Adults should probably limit talking in depth with children about details of the patient's care. For example, there's usually no need to discuss the specific types of medications or the cost of care with a child. Instead, the focus should be on helping the child understand cancer in basic, age-appropriate terms. Of course, the message should be personalized for the individual child and that child's personality, attention span, interests, and life experiences and should be adapted as you talk. For some children, using the metaphor of cancer as a little, imaginary monster might work, but other children might find that analogy either scary or cartoonish, depending on what they know about monsters. Using clear, honest words and phrases usually makes communicating with children easier for both the adult and the child and also more successful for both individuals.

It is also important to keep in mind the child's relationship with the person who has cancer. How well does the child know the patient? Does that person live geographically close, or far away? How will the cancer treatment change childcare or parental visitation? Keeping this relationship in mind will help the adult prepare for potential questions the child might ask during the conversation about the illness or unexpectedly at a later time. Sometimes children immediately wonder how the illness will affect their own day-to-day life, and sometimes that concern arises later, when the child's routine is affected. So a child may ask whether Grandma will still be able to babysit, whether Uncle Joe will live at the hospital, or whether Mom will have to quit her job. Some children are especially concerned about who will care for the patient's pet during treatment. Again, a positive, but honest approach, as well as thinking on your feet when tossed an unforeseen question, will come in handy.

Good communication with children—or with anyone—involves listening as well as conveying information. Individuals tend to focus more on what we will say—our performance in a social interaction—than what we hear. With children, listening is an especially important tool for an adult to use. After the child has a simple explanation of cancer, the adult may opt to wait for at least several seconds before saying more. This pause in conversation can seem excruciating when discussing difficult topics, but it gives the child a little time to process the information and decide how to respond. Asking children how they feel or what questions they have can help them express and seek information so that the adult and child can work toward shared meaning. Often, adults do not to listen attentively to children, but a conversation about cancer is definitely a time not to be too rushed or distracted to listen.

Children tend to ask what they need to know. Their questions will give you useful bits of information so that you can decide what to say—or not say—next. Listen both to *what* they ask and also to *how* they ask it. When faced with information about an adult's illness or death, children can be very direct or blunt, sometimes asking even a healthy parent whether they might die.

Longtime child advocate and creator of his own children's television show, Fred Rogers, suggested that you respond to questions like that with something like, "I hope to be alive for a long, long, long, long time. And no matter what, there will always be someone to take care of you." Sometimes, children shift the conversation's focus to a more comfortable topic such as, *Can I go play now?* The adult should be prepared to respond to whatever questions emerge. Because more questions or concerns will probably come up over time, there exists no need to try to cover all information in a single conversation. Though it is challenging to be patient, both the adult and child may find it helpful if the adult waits until the child has time to ponder the initial cancer conversation. The adult can remain attuned for other opportunities to discuss the topic. Of course, it is a sound principle that communicating with children involves reassuring the child about the known and being honest about the unknown. This principle might well be applied to all communication about the continuum of cancer care.

Finally, adults should watch for behavioral changes in children who know someone with cancer. Younger children may have new emotional outbursts that do not seem directly related to the conversation about cancer but may be an offshoot expression of their confusion or fear. Some children revert to earlier childhood behaviors that they had left behind—perhaps thumb-sucking—but that suddenly emerge as a coping or comforting strategy. Even older children may become clingy or have trouble sleeping after they are told a parent or close relative has cancer. And that parent or relative may have less energy and patience just as the child begs for increased attention. When changes in behaviors are noticed, that may be a good time to open more conversation and to let children know that, while some behaviors may not be acceptable, they are having normal feelings and will always be loved.

Questions children might want to ask about their diagnosis (or adults may want to ask the healthcare provider on the child's behalf):

- What is the name for my cancer?
- Do you know other kids who have this cancer?
- Can someone catch cancer from me like a cold?
- Will I miss school? If so, how much? Will I have to do homework when I miss school?
- Can I play outside? Can I play sports?
- Will I be stuck with a needle? Are there things that will happen that will hurt?

Cancer at Middle Age

Why Me? Who Knows?

Andy Leahy (the author Anna's father) did not expect his intestinal problems at age 48 to be diagnosed as metastatic liver cancer, and he had never considered that his military service might have increased his risk of cancer. When Lynn Greenholdt felt a bump under her skin on her neck in her forties, it did not occur to her that it could be metastatic breast cancer. Madhavi Samala did not think her occasional stomach and bowel upset was colon cancer, several years before a screening *colonoscopy*—a medical procedure to examine the colon—would usually be recommended. Adam Schmitz thought his seizure was more likely a stroke than a brain tumor, but he expected neither in his forties. (Lynn, Madhavi, and Adam were author Anna Leahy's friends.) When cancer sidelined them, they each had pulled together their personal lives and had found jobs they enjoyed. Madhavi and Adam each were raising kids. All their parents were still alive. They had no way to predict they would get cancer at what is a relatively young age.

Neither Amanda Niehaus nor Patricia Grace King expected to hear someone tell them they had breast cancer. Amanda was in her thirties, raising a new daughter, and following her professional interests as a scientist. Patricia was in her forties and on a prestigious yearlong writing fellowship. Patricia considered herself extraordinarily healthy and didn't know other women her age who'd had cancer. They had never thought of themselves at risk, certainly not just when things were going well personally and professionally.

While more than 12% of women in the United States will be diagnosed with breast cancer at some point in their lives, the vast majority of women will never develop breast cancer (NCI, 2016). When Patricia was told by one of her physicians that it was very rare for a woman to be diagnosed with breast cancer in her forties, that was true based on the numbers for her age: a 1.47% chance (NCI, 2016). But there are a lot of women in their forties. Think more broadly—think of how many women in a city like Chicago, where Patricia lived at the time, are in their forties. On average, 1 in every 68 of those forty-something women will be diagnosed with breast cancer. That is a lot of actual middle-aged women with breast cancer.

So, a cancer diagnosis in middle age is rare. But a lot of people still hear that news—that they have cancer—in the prime of life. You may be happily coasting in what breast cancer survivor and author Kelly Corrigan (2008) calls *the middle place*, with a comfortable lifestyle. You may think of your parents as more likely to face cancer than you are in the next few years. Indeed, Corrigan's father was diagnosed with cancer shortly after she was. Or you may be struggling to pull your life together, feeling stuck in a job or relationship, or still figuring things out for the future. Either way, a cancer diagnosis may seem like an interruption, an upheaval, or a catastrophe in the middle of life.

Cancer Prevention and Middle Age

At least one-half of all deaths in the United States can be attributed to preventable behavioral and social factors, such as poor diets, smoking, alcohol use, and poor environmental health conditions. Other first-world nations show similar statistics (NCI, 2016). Behaviors associated with increased risk for cancers have been consistently linked to mortality rates, but oftentimes people do not consider the potentially hazardous outcomes of such behaviors. As we grow older, however, we often realize that our behaviors and lifestyle affect our health and how we feel physically.

We often begin to receive and pay attention to health messaging when we reach our forties. A woman may begin annual mammograms at age 40 or 50, depending on which recommendations she and her general practitioner or gynecologist find right for her. If she has an especially strong family history of breast cancer, as actress Angelina Jolie did, she may opt for genetic testing as part of her assessment of her own risk of developing the disease. Based on that information, Jolie made an unusual decision to undergo a preventative double mastectomy. A person who turns 50 may get a first screening colonoscopy. People in their forties who are still smoking may want to quit more than they did twenty years earlier and may have more willpower. Middle-aged parents may become newly aware of the importance of instilling healthy behaviors in their children. And those diagnosed with cancer in middle age may want to encourage their friends to make healthier choices and avoid behaviors that increase cancer risk.

Health messaging, although most helpful when targeting segmented populations, may be ultimately achieve the highest *efficacy*, or ability to produce desired results, for those in the middle of their lives, old enough to understand the risks, yet young enough to make lifestyle changes that matter. Of course, the earlier we establish healthy behaviors, the lower our risk over the long haul.

Cancer Care and Middle Age

Even if you have lived a relatively healthy life and have a low incidence of cancer in your family, you may still be diagnosed with cancer. Middle age is a time when you are old enough to understand what cancer might mean and actively participate in decisions about your care. In addition, middle-aged patients tend to be healthier than older adults and may have fewer additional health problems, like hearing loss or heart disease, that become more common as we age. In other words, while a cancer diagnosis can be devastating news for a person with children or in the midst of his or her career, a middle-aged person may be in good shape for the widest range of treatment options.

Some people who are in otherwise generally good health when diagnosed with cancer may want to pursue more aggressive or riskier treatment. Younger people may feel as if they have the reserves to tolerate such treatment and much to gain. Every person, of course, is different and weighs the options differently based not only on the cancer diagnosis and prognosis but also on the specific context that includes cultural background, social identity, and physical health.

A person in one's thirties, forties, or fifties, in fact, may have high stakes in a stable social identity. We discuss social identity in Chapter 4 and bring it up here again because middle-aged people may have a well-developed social identity that supports and reinforces their day-to-day lives. If that is the case, these patients are likely to be more concerned about how a cancer diagnosis threatens that established identity than a person whose social identity is in flux. Friends may talk about health problems or changes in their bodies, but a middle-aged person may not know many people their own age who consider themselves sick. Friends may not want to talk about your illness because they do not want to be reminded of the possibility that cancer could happen to them. They may treat you differently, perhaps as if you are more frail than you feel. Though friends and family may be incredibly supportive just when you need it, you may not want to be labeled as *person with cancer*. You may not want to be perceived as *belonging* to that group, just as you have established a strong social identity tied to other categories. So, a cancer diagnosis and treatment may take a toll emotionally and socially in ways that might seem tangential to your physical health and might not be addressed by healthcare professionals.

It may seem strange to talk with a physician or nurse about social identity, but the patient may want to think about ways to seek advice from healthcare providers and perhaps talk with someone who specializes in counseling. When talking with the cancer care team about social identity issues, the patient may feel more comfortable and providers may offer better guidance if the patient connects emotional and social concerns to physical circumstances. For instance, a person in a weekly bridge group may ask whether anything can be done about neuropathy in the hands from chemotherapy that affects the ability to hold a hand of playing cards. A person whose job involves a lot of computer work may have the same concern about neuropathy in the limbs, but for a different reason, a different social identity. A person with a regular golf game may request that radiation treatment be scheduled around that standing social and recreational commitment. Another person may want to schedule appointments around business meetings or childcare. These sorts of conversations allow patients to convey to their healthcare providers what is most important in their lives so that the healthcare providers can understand and work to help the patient maintain the existing social identity. To make the most of these conversations, patients should feel free to express *why* they are concerned—bridge or golf group, job or family obligations—so that an individual's social identity becomes part of the communication about cancer care even when the biomedical information is the priority or at the core of the conversation.

Middle-aged cancer patients also may not have considered how to handle the financial and practical aspects of an illness, and healthcare providers may not be able to address all their patients' practical concerns. Some questions can be addressed by someone in your healthcare organization. How does your healthcare coverage work for a serious or lengthy illness? What kinds of new, perhaps ongoing, expenses might emerge in cancer care that you may have not adequately budgeted? Patients should ask about such concerns. While a physician may know nothing about the billing process or costs, a provider should be able to point the patient to someone in the organization who has information about that issue and that can be used to plan for the future.

Other questions may be ones the patients must answer for themselves. Among family and friends, who might help with care for a few days or a few months? Still other questions should be addressed to an employer, financial advisor, or attorney. If you need to take a medical leave from your job, what is the process for requesting that? Have you named beneficiaries for insurance policies and other financial holdings? Do you have a notarized will? Have you talked with loved ones about the extent of end-of-life care you would want if unexpected circumstances were to arise? *End-of-life*, or the process of dying, brings with it physical, emotional, social, and even legal questions and considerations. It is a good idea for any adult to consider these sorts of questions long before an illness or accident occurs, but we often put off these questions for later in life or until we are forced to face them. A cancer diagnosis often forces a person to address these questions sooner than expected.

If cancer does strike during middle age, patients should know that they are not alone. As the patient makes decisions about health care, stage of life is one of the factors that shapes attitudes and decisions. A patient might consider how to make decisions that give that individual the best possibility for the future life that person wants to have.

Questions adults might want to ask about their diagnosis:

- Will I miss work to undergo treatment? Is there any way to schedule treatment to minimize missed work?
- Does my diagnosis increase the risk my children have of developing this cancer? If so, are there screenings they should undergo now or when they reach my age?
- Will treatment affect my regular routine? Will someone need to drive me to treatments, or can I drive myself? Will my sleep be affected?
- Can I continue to exercising or start exercising? How will cancer and treatment affect my strength and endurance?
- How much will treatment cost me? How does the billing and payment work? If I have employer-based health insurance, does my employer have access to any of my medical information?
- Are there long-term side effects to treatment options? As a result of this diagnosis and treatment, are there health problems I should watch for that might come up in five or twenty years?

Aging and Cancer

Cancer risk correlates with age, so it is no wonder that older adults are diagnosed with cancer at a greater rate than other segments of a population (Berger et al., 2006; Sparks & Nussbaum, 2008). Older adults are considered to be at high risk for poor communication with healthcare professionals (Adelman & Greene, 2000), which can affect cancer care. Older adults have different communicative needs and desires than other age groups, and older adults have unique language, cognitive, physiological, and social issues. All of this will, in some ways, directly and indirectly affect their own health literacy. This, in turn, will have significant implications for the proper care of older cancer patients. In addition, the number and proportion of older adults is growing. The combination of a larger aging population and a higher rate of cancer in that population puts increased demands on the public health system and on medical and social services, of which cancer diagnosis and treatment are a part (Sparks & Nussbaum, 2008). In addition, as we have discussed, people from differing countries or cultures hold differing cultural attitudes toward aging and toward elders. Healthcare providers who are culturally sensitive to the specific needs of older patients facing cancer diagnoses can foster stronger communication with their patients.

According to the World Health Organization (2003), a sharp increase in the number of cancer diagnoses is expected, up from 10 million new cases globally in 2000 to an estimated 15 million in 2020. This rise in cancer diagnoses is due, in large part, to a steady increase in the aging populations in geographical areas across the globe, the continued prevalence of smoking, and the existence of unhealthy lifestyles, which includes poor diets. We are living longer, giving our bodies' cells more time to make the missteps that lead to cancer, and we are not always making healthy choices day to day as we live over decades.

At this time more than any before, those in the healthcare system must work to understand how best to communicate with aging cancer patients across the continuum of cancer care from prevention, detection, and diagnosis to treatment, survivorship, and end-of-life. The study of communication practices during cancer care is now a crucial part of improving *geriatric care*, or care for the elderly (Nussbaum, Baringer, & Kundrat, 2003). Aspects of cancer care that are particular to the aging patient will continue to be increasingly important.

Further, as Sparks and Nussbaum (2008) state, when we age, we face what are called *primary characteristics of aging*, or changes that result solely from the process of growing older. Eventually, for instance, everyone gets wrinkles as a result of altered elasticity because the structure of our skin changes over time. In addition, each individual faces *secondary characteristics of aging*, or changes that occur based on how we live. A lifetime of unhealthy eating, for instance, can cause some individuals to develop diabetes later in life as the long-term effects of a poor diet kick in. In other words, we all face health challenges as we age. Some of them are common to everyone. But some result from our lifestyle choices and do not affect everyone.

Aging and Eyesight

Decline in vision is common as an individual ages, and the first signs often occur around the age of 40. Gradual, age-related decline of the eyes' capacity to focus on close objects, or age-related farsightedness, is known as *presbyopia*. As we age, the eyes' lenses tend to thicken and lose elasticity, and, as a result, we face a slow process of vision loss even if no other conditions, such as cataracts or glaucoma, are present (Corso, 1971; Kline & Scialfa, 1996; McFarland, 1968). It is not uncommon for an individual to cope with such a decline in vision, at least initially, by holding printed material farther from the eyes. By the time a person is 50, small print, details, and even small objects are likely to become more difficult to see, and reading glasses can compensate for that decline in vision. By the age of 70, approximately 70% of the population does not have normal vision even with correction (Botwinick, 1978; Sparks & Nussbaum, 2008). Such eyesight loss due to aging can begin to affect everyday activities.

Older people who are diagnosed with cancer may have trouble reading informational brochures and medication bottles. Such patients should ask questions when they are unable to discern information because of poor eyesight. That said, healthcare providers should explain information verbally and provide information and instructions that they are sure their patients and caregivers can read easily. While that approach should be used for patients of all ages and abilities, providers may need to be particularly aware of ways to ensure their older patients understand information and instructions.

In addition, providers should be attentive to the ways in which poor eyesight could make other symptoms and side effects more painful or dangerous. For instance, a person with poor eyesight may be physically able to climb stairs but may not be able to see stairs well. If that patient then suffers some neuropathy in his or her feet from chemotherapy treatment, stairs might be especially dangerous in ways the patient and caregiver do not fully realize.

Aging and Hearing

The ability to hear, especially high-frequency sounds, and process aural communication is also affected by the aging process. *Presbycusis* is the term used to describe hearing loss associated with aging. As with decline in vision, decline in ability to hear increases measurably beginning in one's late forties, and one out of five people over the age of 75 experiences at least mild hearing loss (Darbyshire, 1984). Even when they think they are hearing correctly, those with the often gradual hearing loss related to aging may be less confident about their own hearing. As a result, they may tend to request information be repeated, curtail conversation, or avoid conversations, especially in a noisy environment.

Older individuals with hearing loss may also try to hide their shortfalls in hearing or overcompensate with tactics such as taking more time to respond, talking over others, or filling silences. Any conversational misstep can be uncomfortable or confusing, so odd or inappropriate fillers in a conversation, especially when it becomes a habit, can be awkward or confusing for all involved in the conversation. Therefore, providers and caregivers of older patients with cancer need to listen for signs that the patient is not hearing well. Such signs might include conversations that do not follow expected norms, the patient seeming to use the wrong words in responses, or the patient responding inappropriately in tone or behavior. Misunderstandings stemming from hearing loss can emerge easily and sometimes subtly and can affect care. In addition, sometimes confused conversations or misunderstanding can lead the provider, caregiver, and patient to think, mistakenly, that cognitive abilities are also diminishing.

Aging and Cognitive Function

Some aspects of cognition slightly decrease as we age, especially after the age of 70 (Anstey & Smith, 1999). Preventative measures such as mental and physical activity throughout the lifespan and especially as we move past middle age can prevent or delay some decline in cognition (Schaie, 1996). Older adults may struggle when making inferences based on information communicated through an interaction more than do younger adults (Nussbaum, Pecchioni, Robinson, & Thompson, 2000; Sparks & Nussbaum, 2008). The older cancer patient may take extra time to figure things out or may strain in ways that raise concerns in others that the patient is not getting the point of the exchange, is confused about a particular point, or is disoriented more generally.

Older adults may struggle with everyday problem-solving as well, sometimes simply because the strategies they have learned and prefer differ from strategies used by younger adults (Nussbaum et al., 2000) Times change, and older adults may be set in the ways they established decades earlier. Older adults can struggle when mentally searching for information, which experts call *declarative cognitive activities*, and when using prior experiential knowledge, which cognitive scientists call *procedural memory and thinking*.

Aging can have positive effects for the individual, too, and can foster certain kinds of wisdom that younger people have not had time to acquire. When performing declarative thinking, older adults often can sift through vast amounts of information and pull out relevant pieces of information necessary for choosing the best option available, whereas younger adults tend to act more like novice searchers by gathering extensive information before sifting through. When performing procedural problem-solving, older adults often rely on their wealth of experiences and well-established strategies for obtaining solutions to the problem. Such strategies may not always adapt well to new circumstances and changing times and may sometimes come across as stubbornness, but tried-and-true ways of approaching life give the older cancer patient a strong foundation on which to rely when deciding what to do.

Aging and Memory

Similar to the research on aging and cognitive abilities, research studying the influence of aging on memory indicates that sensory, short-term, and long-term memory can all be affected by the aging process (Nussbaum et al., 2000; Sparks & Nussbaum, 2008). If a cancer patient is experiencing memory problems, it can help to figure out which kind of memory has been affected in order to help the patient compensate in the most effective ways possible.

Sensory memory is defined as one's ability to process immediately and remember stimuli within a fraction of a second after exposure. When sensory memory is compromised, a patient may have trouble with conversations or instructions. This sort of memory loss may be the easiest for others to notice, which is good. But sensory memory loss may be especially problematic for cancer care because the patient can become confused in the moment or not realize that some information has been missed. A primary caregiver may have to play a bigger role in healthcare decisions, and physicians may need to take extra time to make sure the patient is as fully informed as possible.

Short-term memory is defined as the ability to remember stimuli—a conversation, for instance, or an image—several seconds, minutes, or hours after exposure. If you forget where you parked your car when you come out of the grocery store or forget what you were looking for after you go into a room to look for it, that is a lapse in short-term memory. Most people experience occasional lapses like this, and short-term memory can slowly decline with age. Conversational difficulties tend to arise for older adults when they struggle to simultaneously process sensory stimuli in the moment and also store information as short-term memory. Repetition of information may be helpful during interpersonal communication, and the patient with short-term memory loss may need information written down so that it can be read again later.

Long-term memory refers to experiential or *episodic memory*, to knowledge or what cognitive scientists call *semantic memory*, and to *procedural memory*. Though it can take more time for some older adults to retrieve information from long-term memory, they may retain good episodic memory. That means they may have good narrative recall or tend to remember stories in accurate detail. Older adults, for instance, may remember their health history very well. Other older adults may have diminished episodic memory, which may affect the accuracy of the information they provide about their health history and their ongoing symptoms. If episodic memory is spotty in a patient, physicians and caregivers must work to fill in gaps that affect cancer care.

Older adults may have a wealth of semantic memory from which to draw. Such accumulated knowledge, however, may not have kept up with the changing times. Some older adults may have difficulty acquiring new knowledge as easily as in their younger years, may not want to acquire much new information, or may think that they already know what is best. Cancer, however, is a new situation, so physicians and caregivers may need to explain more to such patients so that they can adapt their knowledge to fit their new circumstances.

Strong procedural memory helps us do common, repeated tasks, such as brushing our teeth or driving to work. If we have good procedural memory, we are able to accomplish tasks when not really thinking about them. That is why a baseball player practices swings and watches video-recordings of good hits; once the process is embedded in his procedural memory, he does not have to think every time he is up to bat about exactly how to position his hands and feet or tell himself to swing at just the right split-second. As a cancer patient develops new routines, those routines, too, become part of procedural memory and should become easier to remember and accomplish. For an older cancer patient with compromised procedural memory, however, it can be difficult to learn new routines even after they are repeated over time. These patients sometimes require every office visit or every dose of medicine to be handled as if it were the first time.

Aging, Cultural Attitudes, and Stereotypes

Aging must be considered in the larger cultural context. In some cultures, older adults are respected, whereas in other cultures, aging carries many negative connotations and is not a welcome stage of life. In the United States, according to research, older adults are often perceived negatively, negative remarks are often directed at them, and they have negative experiences with people in younger age groups (Sparks & Miller-Day, 2014). In Hispanic cultures, on the other hand, older adults tend to be treated with respect and retain greater authority (Sparks & Miller-Day, 2014). In countries such as China and Korea, respect for elders is common, and adult children tend to care for elders (Sparks & Miller-Day, 2014). In such cultures, demonstrating a lack of respect for elders is often perceived as disruptive to cultural and family systems. In addition, when Chinese families immigrate to the United States, for example, the older adults in the family may be forced to fend for themselves like never before as their families acclimate to American customs. Disruptions in the cultural or family system can negatively affect communication and also an individual's health outcomes. The ideas about cultural background, which we presented in Chapter 3, must be considered, therefore, in relation to a patient's age. The older the patient is, the more strongly that person's culture is likely to bear on the patient's lifestyle, priorities, and decision-making during cancer care.

In addition, research has found that people sometimes adjust their behavior to accommodate a stereotype that they hold about another person (Tajfel & Turner, 1986). In other words, some people's behavior reflects a preconceived notion or stereotype of a particular person rather than adjusting to that individual's actual behavior. A physician treating a cancer patient from a different culture or one who is older may speak more slowly or more loudly because the provider may assume that those from other cultures or the elderly will have trouble understanding spoken statements. Moreover, research indicates that the social context in which older adults are encountered is the strongest indicator for how that person will be perceived. Encountering an older person in a hospital or nursing home, for instance, leads to assumptions of impairment, whereas encountering that same person in a vibrant business setting leads someone to think of that person as a competent person (Sparks, 2013).

Further, as Lisa Sparks and Michelle Miller-Day describe this authentic scenario (75-year-old mother), "It is possible for an individual to be ethnically non-Hispanic White/Caucasian, but be culturally Hispanic from growing up in the Mexican border town of Brownsville, Texas" (Sparks & Miller-Day, 2014). Similarly, the intercultural literature often refers to the likelihood of stereotyping based on "face identity" or "ethnic identity" of looking Asian, even when the individual has grown up in the United States speaking English with an American accent and with little or no knowledge of the cultural attitudes or of the original language of their historical or ancestral roots in Korea, Japan, China, Vietnam, or so on. While cultural stereotyping can affect the provider–patient interaction at any patient age, providers and caregivers should consider how their assumptions about an older patient affect the provider–patient interaction in potentially negative ways, inhibit shared meaning, or compromise cancer care.

In sum, appearances may not be what they seem. Healthcare providers and caregivers must be conscious of these tendencies toward positive and negative stereotyping of older adults with cancer and work toward understanding the individual patient based on the patient's attitudes and behaviors.

Aging and Relationships

An older patient's relationships with family and friends may function differently than they have in the past as well as differently than a younger person's relationships. Understanding how relationships function for individuals at different stages of life can help an individual adapt to living with cancer. Caring for older patients can be complicated, and research consistently indicates that interpersonal communication is a central component in effective management of the older patient's care (Sparks, 2013; Sparks & Nussbaum, 2008). As we discussed in earlier chapters, cultural backgrounds, social identities, and interpersonal relationships affect a person's health positively and negatively. Research suggests that, as an individual ages, successful adaptation tends to involve a reduction in social interactions, yet a retaining of the most emotionally supportive relationships (Sparks, 2013). In other words, older adults may have fewer but closer or stronger friendships than younger people. During cancer care, these relationships can help the older patient thrive, leading to better health outcomes.

Questions older adults might want to ask about their diagnosis:

- Does my age affect treatment options?
- What will happen if I choose not to treat this cancer?
- Are there side effects of treatment that are worse for someone my age?
- How do other health conditions I have affect my treatment options and chances that treatment will go well? Are there any interactions between the medications I take for other health conditions and the recommended cancer treatments?
- How will cancer and treatment affect my independence? Will I need a caregiver every now and then, or maybe all the time?
- How does Medicare work when it comes to cancer care? How long can I stay in the hospital, a rehabilitation facility, or hospice under Medicare? Can I schedule multiple tests and treatments on the same day? Will Medicare pay for nursing care at home, if I need it?

Stage of Life and Relationships

Communication plays a crucial role in assessing a patient's mental and physical health, no matter the patient's age. The amount and kind of information that emerges through interactions—between patient and healthcare provider, caregiver, family, or friends—is very much related to the patient's age. Our relationships, the ways we interact, and our priorities and goals change as we move from one stage of life to another. Research indicates that, especially when conveying bad news to a patient, having built a positive relationship with the patient is useful for effective communication in this difficult situation (Sparks, Villagran, Parker-Raley, & Cunningham, 2007). For a physician or caregiver to have that sort of positive relationship with a patient, age and how it plays a role in communication and in mental and physical health must be considered as a factor. A patient's relationships, the ways the patient communicates, and the patient's priorities and goals may even influence whether there will be a positive outcome. Fostering existing interpersonal relationships, therefore, may be especially important after a cancer diagnosis.

Exercise & Discussion

In the Patient's Shoes: A *Thinking Exercise*

1. If you were just diagnosed with cancer, how would you want to be told the news? Consider, for instance, whether you would want to be told by phone as soon as the physician had the diagnosis or in person at an office appointment. Consider whether you would want a family member or friend with you when you receive the news. Consider what kind of language the physician should use.
2. In the days and weeks immediately following the diagnosis, how would you want next steps to follow? What would you want from your provider to help you make decisions and plan for the future?
3. What would you consider a serious misstep by a physician in these interactions about diagnosis and treatment? Under what circumstances would you seek a new physician?
4. How would your needs as a patient in this situation be different if the diagnosis occurred when you were seventy years old? What other physical conditions do you have that would affect your decisions about treatment or the ways your body would respond to treatment?

In the Physician's Shoes: A *Thinking Exercise*

1. If you were a physician sharing a cancer diagnosis with a patient, what would you say? Remember that you might tell this news to patients every day. Consider how much information you would share during the discussion of initial diagnosis. Consider what terminology you are likely to need to define for the patient.
2. What would you say differently depending upon how likely the cancer is to be curable, manageable, or terminal?
3. What would you say differently to a child (and the child's parents) or to an older adult?
4. How would you decide what to say to a patient based on the ways you want to interact with your patient in the future? Consider how to set up the next appointment or procedure.

References

Adelman, R., & Greene, M. (2000). Communication between older patients and their physicians. *Clinics in Geriatric Medicine*, *16*, 1–24.

Anstey, K. J., & Smith, G. A. (1999). Interrelationships among biological markers of aging, health, activity, acculturation, and cognitive performance in older adults. *Psychology and Aging*, *14*, 615–618.

Berger, N., Savvides, P., Kooukian, S. M., Kahana, E. F., Deimling, G. T., Rose, J. H., Bowman, K. F., & Miller, R. H. (2006). Cancer in the elderly. *Transactions of the American Clinical and Climatological Association*, *117*, 147–156.

Botwinick, J. (1978). *Aging and behavior* (2nd ed.). New York, NY: Springer.

Bylund, C. L., Galvin, K. M., Dunet, D. O., & Reyes, M. (2011). Using the Extended Health Belief model to understand siblings' perceptions of risk for hereditary hemochromatosis. *Patient Education and Counseling*, 82, 36–41. doi:10.1016/j.pec.2010.03.009

Corrigan, K. (2008). *The middle place*. New York, NY: Hyperion.

Corso, J. (1971). Sensory processes and age effects in normal adults. *Journal of Gerontology*, *26*, 90–105.

Cruce, M. K. & Stinnet, T. A. (2006). Children with cancer. In Phelps, L. (Ed.), *Chronic health-related disorders in children: Collaborative medical and psycheducational interventions* (pp. 41–55). Washington, DC: American Psychological Association.

Darbyshire, J. (1984). The hearing loss epidemic: A challenge to gerontology. *Research on Aging*, 6, 384–394.

Galvin, K. M., Grill, L. H., Arnston, P. H., & Kinahan, K. E. (2012). Beyond the crisis: *Communication between parents and children who survived cancer.* In F. C. Dickson & L. M. Webb (Eds.), *Communication for families in crisis: Theories, research, strategies* (pp. 229-247). New York, NY: Peter Lang.

Grealy, L. (2003). *Autobiography of a face*. New York, NY: Harper Collins.

Harzold, E., & Sparks, L. (2007). Adult child perceptions of communication and humor when the parent is diagnosed with cancer: A suggestive perspective from communication theory. *Qualitative Research Reports in Communication*, *7*, 67–78.

Kline, D. W., & Scialfa, C. T. (1996). Visual and auditory aging. In J. E. Birren & K. W. Schaie (Eds.), *Handbook of the psychology of aging* (4th ed., pp. 181–203). San Diego, CA: Academic Press.

McFarland, R. (1968). The sensory and perceptual processes in aging. In K. Schaie (Ed.), *Theory and methods in research on aging* (pp. 9–52). Morgantown, WV: West Virginia University Press.

National Cancer Institute. (2016). *Cancer control continuum*. Division of Cancer Control & Population Sciences. Retrieved from https://cancercontrol.cancer.gov/od/continuum.html

Nussbaum, J. F., Baringer, D., & Kundrat, A. (2003). Health, communication, and aging: Cancer and older adults. *Health Communication*, *15*, 185–192. doi:10.1207/S15327027HC1502_6

Nussbaum, J. F., Pecchioni, L., Robinson, J. D., & Thompson, T. (2000). *Communication and aging* (2nd ed.). Mahwah, NJ: Lawrence Erlbaum Associates.

Remy, J. (2008). Pilgrim classic: I, robot. Pilgrim steps. *Pilgrim steps* (Personal Blog). 11 March 2008. Retrieved from http://www.janaremy.com/pilgrimsteps/2008/03/11/pilgrim-classic-i-robot

Remy, J. (2013). There's no word for it…. *Pilgrim steps* (Personal Blog). Retrieved from http://www.janaremy.com/pilgrimsteps/2013/10/18/theres-no-word-for-it/

Robinson, L. L., & Hudson, M. M. (2014). Survivors of childhood and adolescent cancer: Life-long risks and responsibilities. *Nature Reviews Cancer, 14*, 61–70. doi:10.1038/nrc3634

Schaie, K. (1996). Intellectual development in adulthood. In J. E. Birren & K. W. Schaie (Eds.), *Handbook of the psychology of aging* (4th ed., pp. 266–286). San Diego, CA: Academic Press.

Sparks, L. (2013). Health communication and caregiving research, policy, and practice. In R. C. Talley & S. S. Travis (Eds), *Caregiving across the professions: A multi-disciplinary, coordinated perspective*. New York, NY: Springer.

Sparks, L., & Miller-Day, M. (2014). Methodological approaches to eliminating health disparities. In B. Whaley (Ed.), *Research methods in health communication: Principles and application* (pp. 318–336). New York, NY: Taylor and Francis.

Sparks, L., & Nussbaum, J. F. (2008). Health literacy and cancer communication with older adults. *Patient Education and Counseling, 71*, 345–350.

Sparks, L., & Villagran, M. (2008). *La Comunicación en el Cancer: Comunicación y apoyo emocional en el laberinto del cancer*. [English translation: Communication and emotional support in the cancer maze.] Madrid, Spain: Aresta.

Tajfel, H., & Turner, J. C. (1986). The social identity theory of intergroup behavior. In S. Worschel & W. Austin (Eds.), *The social psychology of intergroup relations* (2nd ed., pp. 7–24). Chicago, IL: Nelson-Hall.

World Health Organization (2003). Global cancer rates could increase by 50% to 15 million by 2020. http://www.who.int/mediacentre/news/releases/2003/pr27/en/

· 6 ·

NAVIGATING THE LANDSCAPE

Communication in Cancer Care Organizations

at the doctor's

she asks you to take your clothes off
lie down on the bed
you can paper your nakedness if you wish
the robe is a joke
you both know what you look like

—"at the doctor's" by Ivy Alvarez

Carla Malden had been immersed in her husband's cancer care for months. After he'd been diagnosed with colon cancer, he underwent surgery and chemotherapy, and she was his primary caregiver. During this time, she necessarily became more adept with the language and the landscape of cancer care, which had formerly been unfamiliar to her.

"You learn a lot of new words when you find yourself talking to doctors and nurses," Carla Malden (2011) wrote in her book, *Afterimage*. "They throw them at you as though you've been trained to catch them" (p. 40). Throughout Laurence's diagnosis, treatment, and end-of-life care, Malden and her husband met with all sorts of healthcare professionals in all sorts of healthcare settings. She knew Family Doc, Scary Surgeon Lady, Oncology Man, G.I. Cancer Guru at USC, Dr. City of Hope, a nutritionist at UCLA, Chinese Grand Master, and many nurses and technicians. Every time Laurence's treatment or symptoms changed, they adapted and created a make-do routine, a new normal for themselves.

In addition, Malden had a lot of conversations with healthcare providers over the continuum of cancer care, and the way she viewed these interactions shifted as circumstances changed. She writes, "Scary Surgeon Lady pulled up a chair at the nurses' station and sat with me for half an hour. Push had come to shove, and she was suddenly not scary. She told me about when her father was ill (I don't believe she said dying, but I can't remember for sure) and required hospice care. I startled at the word. She told me what it entailed, how it worked" (p. 170). The surgeon who had been off-putting earlier in the cancer care continuum became a helpful matter-of-fact resource later in the experience.

Malden (2011) was negotiating the cancer care continuum as if it were a landscape of new places, people, and terminology, and she was doing pretty well. In fact, even before her husband's surgery, she realized, "I knew that the cancer had not just changed our life; it had changed who I was as well" (p. 84). In this statement, she is expressing the sorts of issues Chapter 4 raises about social identity. At some level, Malden recognized that she and her husband would never return to their old normal because they had been changed as people by the experience of cancer.

In many ways, she was the ideal, aware, active caregiver, an exceptionally adept partner in Laurence's health care. Chapter 8 will discuss the role of caregivers like Carla to a much greater extent. Without previous training, Malden had to coordinate the whole process of care for her husband—visiting nurses, pharmacy deliveries, appointments—and communicate with a variety of experts about a variety of details. Understanding the larger healthcare system is important so that patients and caregivers can make informed decisions, seek support, and prepare for the future. Health communication cannot be fully understood without taking into account the context of healthcare organizations and the ways in which the interactions within healthcare organizations reflect and shape the social reality of cancer care and the individual patient's decision-making.

The Healthcare System

The healthcare system involves many different entities, from a local doctor's office to a regional hospital and, in some countries, to national research facilities. Despite its sometimes large size and multiple components, a healthcare system faces a monumental task in trying to deliver adequate care to everyone who needs care. Poorly coordinated communication, for instance, is sometimes related to problems such as high provider turnover rates (Sparks & Villagran, 2010). Because of its complexity, coordinated communication can be difficult to achieve in such a complex system, even though improved communication among various researchers, providers, and the public could alleviate some problems in delivering adequate care.

Cancer care is part of this larger healthcare system in which there are several bosses, several sets of rules, several different financial charges for the same item, and several different procedures for the same task. The general practitioner's—or family doctor's—office is one organization in this system. In many places, it occupies a set physical space, employs medical and office staff, and has established its own rules, habits, and chain of command. This physician can refer patients to other physicians in different specializations, including oncologists and surgeons for the cancer patient, and to a hospital, which has a different organizational structure, of which the doctor(s) and patient become a part. Each of the three parties—the hospital, the doctor's office(s), and the patient—will communicate directly with the other two, and each will need to relay information to the third party when they get information from that second party. In addition, other entities, such as a laboratory or an outpatient center, will be involved in this interconnected structure and communication process. Sounds confusing. Indeed, these structures and the communication that occurs within and among them can be confusing for anyone, especially a cancer patient who is undergoing physically and mentally demanding therapy. That is why health communication plays an important role in helping patients navigate the healthcare organizations in the cancer care continuum.

Specialists may be involved in a patient's care. Most cancer patients in the United States are treated by a physician called an *oncologist*, who specializes in or focuses entirely on treating cancer. The oncologist's office usually has a similar structure to that of a general practitioner's office but has established its own version of a doctor's office, which often includes an infusion suite in which several patients at once can be given chemotherapy. Patients who undergo surgery are treated by a surgeon and sometimes see a cardiologist before the surgical procedure. In addition to the patient's primary care physician, these other physicians, such as the surgeon and cardiologist, add useful expertise to cancer care but complicate the communication process for an individual patient. The patient, for instance, may need to ensure that each specialist has diagnostic test results and examination records from the other physicians involved in care, sometimes physically carrying records to an appointment.

Multiple hospitals may be involved in care as well. In the United States, patients in need of hospitalization usually go to one relatively nearby. But a patient with cancer may travel to one of the larger cancer centers, such as MD Anderson in Houston, Barnes in St. Louis, Johns Hopkins in Baltimore, Cleveland Clinic, City of Hope in California, or the Mayo Clinic in Minnesota. That is precisely what journalist Christopher Hitchens (2012) did after he was diagnosed with esophageal cancer, the same cancer that had killed his father. He spent time in a hospital in Washington, DC, where he lived, but also received radiation treatment away from home at MD Anderson. In fact, his first inkling that he might have cancer came when he thought he was having a heart attack while promoting his latest book; he was in New York, so he went to a hospital there.

In addition to doctors and hospitals, another important entity is part of the large group of communicators as well: the person or group who is responsible for payment of the expenses related to cancer care. Whether care is being paid for out of pocket by the patient, by an insurance company via a private or employer-based policy, or through a publicly financed program such as Medicare and Medicaid in the United States, the entity that pays the bills will exert constraints on what type of care is allowable for coverage in the program. The type of payment will also determine how much providers can charge for their services, which services are covered in given circumstances, and how much of the cost the patient will bear. Payment for procedures or medications that are deemed to be experimental, for example, sometimes fall heavily on the patient unless the patient is part of a formal research study. All of these issues will need to be communicated to the patient before treatment begins and as it continues, usually by office or hospital staff trained in the process of making payment claims, rather than those recommending or administering treatment. Patients may be focused on questions about their physical well-being and should be aware that questions related to the cost of care and their financial situations are appropriate to ask as part of living the best life possible.

All of these healthcare entities or hubs can create a seemingly chaotic landscape or culture for the patient and a bureaucratic system that occasionally results in miscommunication among parties involved. The patient and oncologist may have a strong relationship built on trust and clear, honest communication, but the specialized nature of cancer and the complexity of the healthcare system make coordinated communication a challenging and very important part of successful cancer care for each individual patient.

Patient Socialization and Cancer Care

When a patient is diagnosed with cancer, this person becomes socialized into the cancer care process or cancer culture over time, just as an individual is socialized into any other system or social structure. When someone goes off to college, joins a church community, or moves to a new country, the person becomes socialized into that new environment. (You can read more about social identity, culture, and socialization in Chapters 3 and 4.) The individual patient must gain and negotiate relevant information about how to navigate cancer care and its organizations.

Organizations do not exist without human interaction and, in fact, are formed and reformed through ongoing interactions between patients and providers. As you become socialized into cancer care, it can be helpful to think about how to handle your new role of self-advocacy for effective cancer treatment, how to learn the roles of other players on your cancer care team, and how to adapt each organization's goals and behaviors to match your own goals and values. Health communication and its understanding of socialization can guide patients.

It may be useful to recognize the three phases of socialization and to consider where the patient is in the process. At the time of diagnosis, for instance, you are unlikely to have your bearings or even realize that *socialization*—the process of learning to behave in ways appropriate to the context—is beginning. As you become socialized into cancer care, a patient will be better able to communicate with the providers, be better at navigating healthcare organizations, and be better equipped to make decisions about next steps in treatment.

Anticipatory Phase

Cancer patients in the *anticipatory phase* of socialization acquire general information, either actively or by happenstance, and form opinions and expectations about the larger healthcare system and about specific health organizations, such as a doctor's office or a hospital. A woman who feels a lump in her breast and schedules a mammogram may browse the Internet for information about breast cancer and the reliability of mammograms, as she prepares herself to become a patient. Making the initial diagnostic appointment and accessing directions to get to the facility are practical steps in socialization.

The anticipatory phase may vary by age, gender, geography, and other factors. A child, like Lucy Grealy at age nine, may look forward to the hospital as a vacation from school. When Grealy (2003) was told that she would have surgery, she did not understand the doctor's terminology or what surgery entailed, so she shared her exciting news at school. "I told my teachers and all of my friends, probably with pride: I had a malignancy. I was going to have a *big* operation now" (p. 43). Lucy reacted as a schoolchild, not as the patient she would become over the ensuing weeks, months, and years. A woman who is scheduled for a diagnostic mammogram may seek advice from a friend who has gone through the diagnostic step in breast cancer care, whether or not that friend was diagnosed with cancer. The anticipatory phase of socialization focuses on gathering information and aligning expectations.

Organizational Entry

The second phase of socialization, *organizational entry*, begins with early interactions the patient has with a healthcare organization. You discover where to park, where to check in, where to wait, perhaps where to wait again—basic navigational information about the environment. You also figure out who's who—who has information about scheduling appointments, who has information about billing, who asks which types of questions and wants what kind of information. You may be given or ask for brochures, video-recordings, website links, and other informational materials. Organizational entry is a phase in which more specific information is gathered and more interaction occurs.

Susan Gubar (2012) describes part of her organizational entry early in *Memoir of a Debulked Woman*. At first, she did not have symptoms that struck her as serious, so she was not aware that she should be seriously concerned. Digestive problems and feeling full sent her to the hospital. There, she met the *hospitalist*, a physician who works only with patients in the hospital and, in her case, the person who read Gubar's CT scan in the Emergency Room. That is when her relationship with a healthcare organization shifted more dramatically, and she began gathering information specific to the cancer care continuum. "Then and there, a doctor hastily processed papers for admission to the hospital—presumably to get me quickly to an oncologist" (Gubar, 2012, p. 5). Often, when cancer is suspected, the patient becomes quickly drawn into the healthcare system. That shift may cause anxiety and uncertainty, or it might come as a relief, a sense of increased understanding, or a sense of being well taken care of. Gubar (2012) felt something like freedom or euphoria in the moments after diagnosis and recalls, "I remember a moment of extraordinary calm when left on a gurney with a whisper of the initial diagnosis of advanced ovarian cancer" (p. 5).

As in Susan Gubar's case, a cancer diagnosis is often not expected, even if the patient has the sense that something is physically wrong. When a biopsy is scheduled, perhaps following a mammogram or an abdominal x-ray, a patient knows that cancer is a possibility but usually hopes there is some other explanation. Some patients have a sense that something is very wrong and feel some relief that the cause of their symptoms has been discovered and named. Many patients do not experience this moment of calm in the moments immediately following, especially because they are often in the unfamiliar environment of a hospital or a doctor's office and not fully socialized into the cancer care system. A cancer diagnosis may be the cause of organizational entry but can also make socialization into the organization challenging because the days following diagnosis are often stressful.

Assimilation

When a cancer patient gains a fuller understanding of the diagnosis and treatment options and when that individual becomes an active participant in patient–provider communication about next steps and healthcare decisions, that patient has assimilated to the cancer care system. The patient then begins to align personal goals, values, and expectations with those of others in the organization. This phase of socialization is one of adjustment and acclimation in which the patient moves from being an outsider to being an insider.

Assimilation, then, is sense-making. The patient makes sense of the cancer care surroundings and circumstances based on communication, action, and interpretation. Out of what may initially seem like an enormous, chaotic healthcare environment, the patient uses communication to bring order to and create a reality for ongoing cancer care. A specific patient's cancer care team does not really exist in this specific iteration before that person is diagnosed with cancer, so the reality is indeed created in real time as the patient socializes into cancer care.

In her book *In the Body of the World,* playwright and activist Eve Ensler (2013) describes her visit to the Mayo Clinic, a place she calls "Cancer Town":

> Everyone knows that everyone who comes there is finding out if they're sick, already sick, getting better from being sick, or too sick and will probably die. The whole town is like one palliative care unit. The waitresses are grief counselors. They serve you hamburgers and hold your hand as you weep [...]. All the sales people, the street cleaners, the airport shuttle drivers have an eye out for the wounded. There are wig stores on every corner. (p. 21)

Whether "cancer town was a comfort or a horror" (Ensler, 2013, p. 22), being there forced her—and many others seeking diagnosis and treatment—to assimilate to the cancer care continuum.

Though you would certainly rather not be part of the cancer care system, you often do not have much choice once you have actually faced a cancer diagnosis. Moreover, you often do not feel a lot of control over the pace at which the organization encourages you to assimilate. Poet and cultural critic Meghan O'Rourke (2011) talks about what psychiatrists call *numbing out;* she temporarily shut down her emotions as she continued to intellectually process new information about the progression of her mother's colorectal cancer. Even at the Mayo Clinic, Ensler (2013) felt as if she were in "a kind of trance" (p. 23) and wished she could disappear from the examining table. But just a few days later, after she had assimilated more fully, she learned from a tough-love nurse how to care for her own stoma, the new hole in her body. Being aware of where you are in the socialization process can help you pace your decisions. A patient will make more informed, confident decisions once that person assimilates and is more knowledgeable about cancer care, the specific cancer situation, and the role of a patient working with a team of healthcare professionals within the larger system.

In some cases, savvy cancer patients can change from an unsatisfactory cancer system to one that is a better fit for the patient and family members in terms of communicating messages of hope and resilience in more effective ways during the treatment process. It is important to know that one size does not fit all patients and family members and that the organizational system of choice can be a very personal one. The outcome and treatment options within each system and across systems may be similar, but the process and delivery of cancer care can be vastly different. We often have choices and, with some effort, can enact those choices if needed and desired for obtaining the best cancer care experience.

Healthcare Organizations and Learning

Because healthcare organizations are made up of the many people who inhabit them, they can be said to *learn*. The organization can shift as information is exchanged within its system and with the larger environment. The organization can adapt itself from one patient to the next, forming a different team and treatment protocol as each patient enters the organization. And that team and protocol for a specific patient can be adapted as circumstances change, whether that be a cancer-free body that requires follow-up care, progression of the disease, debilitating side effects of chemotherapy, or a change in who is responsible for payment. All of this responsiveness, of course, requires clear, efficient communication of information.

Based on work by Peter Senge (1990), communication experts consider five disciplines, or organizational skills, to be important in achieving organizational adaptability. We consider and have adapted how these skills apply to the cancer patient.

Systems Thinking

Systems thinking is the ability to consider and improve connections and patterns within systems as a whole. Organizations with weak systems thinking often cannot see the forest for the trees; they lose sight of the big picture and fail to see the structural complexity that is present. When all parties who are part of a patient's cancer care team keep the larger picture in mind and do not get bogged down by a particular detail and do not become isolated, they are able to work well in coordinating and sharing goals.

Individual Mastery

When each person who is involved in the care of a cancer patient—physician, nurse, technician, social worker, billing agent—spends a great deal of time learning their specific craft and keeping up with new practices in their field, the organization is said to have personal or *individual mastery*. Each person knows a specific role well and also takes time to understand how that role relates to the roles of others caring for that patient.

Mental Models

Mental models are deeply engrained assumptions, generalizations, and images of how a process, such as cancer care, works. These mental models are often unstated and must be learned through socialization into the organization. Mental models can provide stability and efficiency for an organization. However, because communication about mental models is often weak, organizations can run into problems when, without anyone realizing it, not every individual has exactly the same assumptions or generalizations about an aspect of cancer care.

Mental models can be especially difficult for patients to discern. When young Lucy Grealy was told she would undergo chemotherapy once a week and that it would be given by injection, she assumed that the experience would be just like getting the shots she'd had before surgery. She had a mental model for *injection*, but she did not have a mental model for *chemotherapy* and could not know that her healthcare providers and even her parents carried in their heads assumptions about the experience that differed from her own.

In addition, over-reliance on existing mental models can make organizations inadvertently resistant to opportunities, new treatment protocols based on recent research, and cutting-edge technology. It is easy for any organization to fall into habitual ways of doing things because of routine. Revising mental models can be difficult for an organization to do unless the mental model it has of itself includes the notion that it is agile. And revising mental models is impossible without strong, clear, efficient communication across parts of the organization.

Shared Vision

Mental models help establish a *shared vision*, or common idea the cancer care team creates and shares regarding the future. Ideally, the shared vision is to guide the patient through treatment with the goal that the patient will become a long-term survivor. While this shared vision is sometimes unrealistic, it often leads each person who is involved in the care of a cancer patient—physician, nurse, technician, social worker, billing agent—to excel and to work hard toward the common goal. Organizations that encourage shared vision motivate their employees, and this encouragement is achieved through strong communication.

Team Learning

Learning always begins with communication. *Team learning* occurs when everyone on the cancer care team works together to create the conditions for learning to occur by communicating information efficiently and clearly throughout the team. The patient receives the best care when the healthcare professionals caring for that person adapt together as they administer care.

Hospice as Coordinated Communication and Whole-Patient Care

Hospice is a healthcare organization that works in concert with other organizations, including the doctor's office, the hospital, and the pharmacy, to provide care for the terminally ill. Hospice is an increasingly important part of the continuum of cancer care. As the opening chapter of *Communication at the End of Life* (Nussbaum, Giles, & Worthington, 2015) points out:

> As health care has improved, more and more individuals are aware of the impending terminality of themselves and those around them. As people are living longer, more of us ultimately die of something anticipated. The issues relating to communication *with* those who are dying and the communication *of* those who are dying have become increasing[ly] relevant both personally and in the literature of health communication as a result. (Thompson, 2015, p. 12)

Hospice care addresses this reality that many cancer patients face and incorporates individuals' awareness of terminality into care and communication about illness and well-being at the end of life.

A hospice, which we will discuss in Chapter 8 as well, is sometimes housed within a hospital or in a stand-alone facility, or hospice services can be offered in the patient's home. Regardless of the location, the goal of hospice care is to encourage a distinctive environment to support terminally ill patients and their families. The organization uses coordinated communication to improve the quality of life in a patient's final months or days. To achieve this, hospice workers—healthcare professionals and volunteers—are specially trained, and care focuses on the whole patient, especially on managing pain, stress, and suffering.

Communication within a hospice organization and between hospice and other healthcare entities takes into account the physical, social, and spiritual needs of a patient. The hospice nurse assigned to a patient will work directly with the treating physician and the pharmacy to provide useful care and medication and will train the caregivers in its administration. Often, hospice can arrange for a hospital bed at home or for a volunteer to wash the patient's hair. Hospice can also arrange for spiritual support, perhaps a minister or a lay person trained in religious grief counseling. In hospice, communication is centralized, agile, and honest.

Resistance and Acceptance

Given her intense experience over months, it is difficult to imagine that Carla Malden (2011) could be any more prepared for end-of-life decisions. When a scan revealed that her husband's colorectal cancer had spread to the liver, the physician's tone changed, and he presented pain management, not going after the cancer, as the top priority. Not only was Malden as prepared as she could have been through her experience, but the oncologist also made a clear statement that Laurence was probably not going to get better. After all that, when she heard the word *hospice*, she was still taken by surprise.

"Looking back at it now," Malden (2011) wrote, "I cannot believe we couldn't manage to process the subtext. I couldn't anyway. Or refused to" (p. 103). What the oncologist had said, of course, was not complicated subtext. It was only later, however, when Laurence was back in the hospital and his health was more obviously declining, that Carla understood what was going on. For her, the word *hospice* opened up a new terrain in the landscape of cancer care. Looking back on it as she wrote her book, Malden (2011) realized that the caregiving she had been doing was already their "own version of hospice" (p. 144).

Like Carla Malden, who was startled by the word *hospice* even though she knew her husband's prognosis was not good, Mary Lee Leahy (the mother of one of this book's authors) bristled when her oncologist mentioned that it was time to consider hospice. Though she had not expected to live more than a year after diagnosis (and this was about eight months into cancer care), her initial thought in response to her oncologist's suggestion was akin to *Not yet—I'm not that bad yet*. In addition, though she had known people in hospice care, she had lingering notions of what hospice meant from decades earlier and imagined a bed-ridden, heavily drugged person who had taken a sudden turn for the worse and needed immediate, constant attention, not someone who could sit in her doctor's office and hold a conversation. Her family encouraged her to try hospice, in part because they could not provide the level of care themselves that the oncologist explained hospice would be able to deliver at home. As soon as hospice swooped in, Mary Lee felt well attended and more comfortable, emotionally and physically, as the center of attention, with necessary drugs on hand and a specially designed air mattress. Her caregivers felt as if they were better supported, with information or assistance just one phone call away at any time.

Back-and-forth communication between the hospice workers and caregivers is crucial in order to avoid misinterpretation and address any disagreement about the course of care. Hospice workers must take into account the lack of expertise that many caregivers have for specific tasks and also must be responsive to a caregiver's concern that the patient is overmedicated, as Robin Romm (2009) wrote in *The Mercy Papers* about her mother's hospice care, or not receiving enough medication to alleviate pain or agitation.

Hospice is an exemplar among healthcare organizations, but hospice is *not* for all cancer patients. Sometimes doctors do not discuss hospice services until the patient asks about them, so the patient or family member may want to initiate this important discussion if the prognosis is dire or if the patient's decline is significant and steady. Below are some questions the patient or family might ask the provider about hospice services if it becomes appropriate to consider hospice as an option for care.

- When is a patient eligible for hospice? Who decides?
- When is the right time for me (or my family member), given this type and stage of cancer, to start thinking about hospice care?
- Are there inpatient facilities in this area? Is home hospice care available in this area?
- Is there anything I need to do to prepare for hospice?
- Will a constant caregiver be needed if I choose to use hospice services?
- What about times when my doctor is unavailable? Are hospice workers in charge of my medical care?
- What kinds of palliative care are provided by hospice?
- What kinds of treatment are limited by hospice? If I feel well enough, can I leave the house even if I am using hospice services?
- Are there any additional costs for hospice care?

Limits of Hospice as an Organization

As comprehensive as hospice care can be, hospice does not take care of every possible need for every patient and family. Some patients and caregivers may need and be able to afford supplemental services not provided by hospice, such as a night nurse. Robin Romm (2009) and her father had hospice care but realized, "Trading nights with Mom has everyone feeling frail. We need to hire a nurse" (p. 153). Hospice is a hub organization and can provide a list of nursing providers and other resources not directly provided by hospice itself.

In the final weeks, Mary Lee, too, had some additional nursing care despite the expense. The family contacted a home healthcare agency that hospice recommended and hired a licensed practical nurse, or LPN, for an occasional day or night shift, depending on the caregivers' schedules and levels of exhaustion. Mary Lee was especially comforted by a tiny yet strong woman who could turn her without causing discomfort and who sang to her as she rubbed lotion onto her arms and legs. This nurse was able to communicate useful information about Mary Lee's physical state directly to the family and to hospice workers when they were present at the same time, so that, even though she did not work directly for the hospice organization, her participation in care was coordinated as well.

While not every family can afford additional paid care, inviting comforting individuals into the environment can be helpful—physically, emotionally, and even socially—to the patient, the family, and those who have been caregivers over time.

Organizational Benefits

With hospice care, the patient and family become less burdened by logistics like phone calls, appointments, and errands. They can shift their focus to making the most of their time together and dealing with the grief they are feeling. The information about end-of-life that hospice provides and the supportive care can allow patients and families to communicate more openly about a variety of topics among each other and also with trained professionals. Hospice tends to reduce the stress that a terminal illness causes. In fact, some research indicates that patient preferences may shift during the cancer process. Further, terminally ill patients may end up living longer in hospice care, sometimes well beyond a physician's prognosis or longer than do terminally ill patients who continue aggressive treatment (Balaban, 2000; Wright, Sparks, & O'Hair, 2013).

Although no amount of communication can change the outcome for some cancer patients, effective communication in which various healthcare providers, volunteers, and caregivers effectively balance the cancer care tasks and relationships leads to situations in which patients and the healthcare team are more team oriented, more satisfied with their time and effort, and ultimately more successful at maximizing the potential of health care (Sparks, 2013). Hospice is an exemplar among healthcare organizations in the larger healthcare system because care is well coordinated and all individuals tend to work toward shared goals.

Exercise & Discussion

This exercise asks you to empathize with people in different circumstances as you consider how patients assimilate into the healthcare system. Prior experience with the healthcare system varies among individuals, and socialization into a healthcare organization can be easier or more difficult depending on that prior experience. Discuss how the following experiences or backgrounds might affect a person's socialization that follows a cancer diagnosis.

- Your aunt is a surgeon.
- Your mother is a nurse in a physician's office.
- You have a fear of needles.
- You are allergic to latex.
- You have never taken a sick day from school or work.
- One of your parents died of cancer.
- You are (or want to become) a physician.
- You have not had a checkup in twenty years.
- You have diabetes—or hemophilia or heart disease.
- You live more than 50 miles from the closest city and hospital.
- You are a single parent of school-age children.
- You were diagnosed and treated for a different cancer more than ten years ago.
- The cancer you have is a recurrence of the same one you thought had been treated successfully several years earlier.
- You have not had positive experiences with your primary care physician.

References

Balaban, R. B. (2000). A physician's guide to talking about end-of-life care. *Journal of General Internal Medicine, 15*, 195–200.

Ensler, E. (2013). *In the body of the world*. New York, NY: Metropolitan.

Grealy, L. (2003). *Autobiography of a face*. New York, NY: Harper Collins.

Gubar, S. (2012). *Memoir of a debulked woman*. New York, NY: W.W. Norton.

Hitchens, C. (2012). *Mortality*. New York, NY: Twelve (Hachett).

Malden, C. (2011). *Afterimage: A brokenhearted memoir of a charmed life*. Guilford, CT: Skirt.

Nussbaum, J. F., Giles, H., & Worthington, A. (Eds.). (2015). *Communication at the end of life*. New York, NY: Peter Lang.

O'Rourke, M. (2011). *The long goodbye*. New York, NY: Riverhead.

Romm, R. (2009). *The mercy papers: A memoir of three weeks*. New York, NY: Scribner.

Senge, P. (1990). *The fifth discipline: The art & practice of learning organization*. New York, NY: Doubleday.

Sparks, L. (2013). Health communication and caregiving research, policy, and practice. In R. C. Talley & S. S. Travis (Eds.), *Multidisciplinary, coordinated caregiving* (pp. 131–176). New York, NY: Springer.

Sparks, L., & Villagran, M. (2008). *La Comunicación en el Cancer: Comunicación y apoyo emocional en el laberinto del cancer*. [English translation: Communication and emotional support in the cancer maze.] Madrid, Spain: Aresta.

Thompson, T. (2015). Health communication and death studies. In J. F. Nussbaum, H. Giles, & A. Worthington (Eds.), *Communication at the end of life* (2nd ed., pp. 11–26). New York, NY: Peter Lang.

Wright, K. B., Sparks, L., & O'Hair, H. D. (2013). *Health communication in the 21st century* (2nd ed.). Oxford: Blackwell.

· 7 ·

WHAT'S UP, DOC?

Patients and Healthcare Providers in Conversation

A wizened face replaces
    the soft gentle dew
    of youth.

Fading memories of a week
    ago when you lay dying
    and I wanted to help you
        but couldn't

and I wanted to help take the
pain away
    but couldn't

and wanted to take you
    in my...
        in my arms
            but couldn't.

—from "The Music Box" by Frank L. Meyskens, Jr.

Kelly Corrigan wanted the physician who read her mammogram films to recognize her panic and alleviate her worries. She became so stressed out as he stood in front of the lightbox displaying images of her breasts that she started grinding her teeth. Her physician wanted a biopsy quickly, but Corrigan was struggling to prioritize her questions and couldn't process all of the information at once.

Kelly Corrigan's (2008) physician said that he was "very concerned about the—well, the mass" (p. 24). He pointed to the image of her breast and told her that he was scheduling her for a core needle biopsy that week. She tried to take in all the information quickly, including the size of the mass. The physician used the word *explosion* to describe it. One can imagine that such language, along with a cancer diagnosis, would be startling to most patients. Corrigan (2008) was very aware that this provider–patient interaction was uncomfortable for both of the individuals involved. She recalls in her memoir *The Middle Place*, "I can see my reaction is making Dr. White uneasy but not so uneasy that he offers up any hope. He doesn't say 'Oh, I see I have alarmed you…' He doesn't say 'Don't get ahead of yourself.' He doesn't say 'Many times, these mammogram films are misleading'" (p. 24). In the moment, the physician does not tell the patient what she expects to hear or wants to hear, and he certainly does not seem to realize this communication failure.

Corrigan was not able to process all the information she heard and saw during this interaction with her provider, in part because she did not understand what some of the terminology meant. "I'd like to know what 'core needle' is," Corrigan (2008) writes, "but I'm more interested in why he's 'concerned'" (p. 24). She was working hard to think clearly but also, of course, had an emotional response to the fact that she had breast cancer and that the tumor was larger than she had imagined. "I feel like a four-year-old who has just spun around in the grocery store and realized that the woman she thought was her mother is a stranger and every aisle she looks down is empty and every voice she hears is the wrong one. Red hot tears start streaming down my cheeks" (p. 24). She left the appointment upset and still trying to figure out what she felt and what questions she had.

Corrigan's brain latched on to specific phrasing the radiologist has used, words that she repeated later to her husband and mulled over as she worried and waited for the next step, words like *very concerned*, *explosion*, *tentacles*. Even by the time she talked with her husband on the phone, she was already comparing her seven-centimeter tumor to a colleague's one-centimeter tumor and wondering what that difference might mean for her prognosis. She was actively thinking through as much as she could, but the communication with her healthcare provider had left her reeling.

Dr. White, whom Corrigan found staid and too comfortable in what was an uncomfortable situation for her, was not this patient's general practitioner, nor was he the oncologist who would treat her for cancer. He had a very limited role in the process of Corrigan's care, but his role placed him at a crucial point—diagnosis—in the conversation about cancer. His goal was to make sure that his patient understood the next step: she had to come back for a needle biopsy, which he had scheduled for that Friday. Dr. White undoubtedly wanted to treat the interaction as a professional one and to focus on the biomedical reality of the situation. It sounds as if he did not view the next step in cancer care as Corrigan's decision.

Often, an interaction between a patient and a provider achieves the provider's top goal, as it did in this instance. Sometimes, that suffices for the patient as well. It is not possible for all patient–provider interactions to be comprehensive, nor is it always beneficial to try to achieve both breadth and depth in a given conversation. Still, how each conversation unfolds affects the overall cancer care process. As we discuss in this chapter, patients and providers can improve their communication in distinct ways, which, in turn, will enrich their sense of well-being and their ability to make decisions together with shared meaning. Understanding goals and motivations of both providers and patients in cancer communication is crucial to analyzing and optimizing decision-making throughout the continuum of cancer care.

Talking with Healthcare Providers: Three Aspects of Communication

Healthcare providers can be the primary source of reliable information about treatment options and prospects for recovery at every stage in the cancer care process. Physicians, physician assistants, nurse practitioners, nurses, social workers, and laboratory technicians play significant roles in communicating with a patient about cancer, and they are valuable members of a healthcare team. While healthcare providers have the knowledge and experience to answer many questions about the illness, they rarely anticipate and fulfill all, or even most, of a patient's informational, emotional, and psychological needs. In general, provider–patient communication has three major aspects or functions. Understanding these aspects will help you strengthen and balance them in provider–patient interactions.

In fact, patients may want to share this chapter, if not this whole book, with their physicians. The patient is the most important person in cancer communication, and we hope that physicians, other healthcare providers, caregivers, and family and friends will find the information in this book useful in their interactions with patients. After all, we're conversing with cancer together as individuals, organizations, and communities. The field of health communication recognizes this complex, interconnected system of interaction.

Control

The first aspect or function of communication between a patient and cancer care providers is *control*. Every formal interaction in our lives establishes so-called rules of engagement. In other words, interaction between a patient and a healthcare provider follows unstated principles about how we are supposed to interact in that particular situation. The roles for patients and providers draw from conventional cultural norms, including our assumptions about well-trained, white-coated physicians. But these roles are negotiated from the very first meeting between individuals and throughout the cancer care process.

In typical provider–patient interactions, the provider has control over the flow of information because the provider asks most of the questions and then doles out information on topics related to that patient's care, often focusing on the single next step. Because they have access to the means for saving lives and alleviating illness and pain, physicians traditionally have a significant amount of power in interactions with patients. For this reason, a patient often feels at a disadvantage when talking with a surgeon or an oncologist, especially after hearing about a cancer diagnosis.

Although patients cannot choose to not have cancer—cannot alter the situation or context for the interaction—they can play a major role in the way their communication with cancer care providers occurs. Each interaction with a provider is negotiated in real time, not set in stone. Patients and providers come to each visit with a set of needs for information and a set of objectives or goals. Patients share control over how information is exchanged and how the relationship is created and maintained.

A formal relationship between a doctor and patient is likely to start out as very structured, with the provider managing the types of topics discussed and the flow of communication. Over time, however, control may rebalance, especially if the patient actively engages in communication that shifts the balance. The interactions may become less structured or involve more give-and-take between the provider and patient about realistic objectives and treatment options. As the patient becomes more familiar with medical terminology and what is happening to to the patient's own body, the patient may carry more of the conversation, ask more questions, and bring additional information to bear on the interaction. As the relationship progresses, patients tend to have more control over communication; they share in decision-making and topic selection for interactions. Over time, many patients are able to freely discuss various topics with their providers, seek more complex information, and voice concerns about their treatment options, current physical state, or progress. Those patients who remain uncomfortable may want to bring a family member or friend who is able to engage more overtly or openly with healthcare providers over time.

Affiliation

Another aspect of the provider–patient relationship is *affiliation*, which refers to our aspiration or need to build a mutually respectful relationship based on humanity and dignity. Research suggests most people value competence over friendliness in their physicians and, if they had to choose, would opt for a highly competent but unfriendly physician than a very friendly but not very skilled physician (Sparks & Villagran, 2010), so affiliation may not seem to be the most important function for a patient or a provider. However, healthcare providers who build strong interpersonal relationships with patients are less likely to face malpractice lawsuits, which suggests that building rapport is important in very practical terms for the doctor as well as for the patient (Levinson et al., 1997; Huntington & Kuhn, 2003; Sparks & Villagran, 2010; Wright, Sparks, & O'Hair, 2013). For example, when Kelly Corrigan (2008) wanted Dr. White to offer comforting words to alleviate her panic, this stemmed from her need for kindness. Dr. White, however, did not recognize that a more personal exchange could benefit himself as well as his patient in the long run, especially if he were ever to make a mistake in his diagnostic process.

The most effective provider–patient relationships are those in which communication is used to show kindness, build trust, and demonstrate mutual respect as well as to share information and goals. Affiliation increases when patients feel they can connect with their providers as people over the length of their relationship, which may extend months or years through cancer treatment and follow-up care. Therefore, the responsibility for affiliation falls most heavily on the healthcare provider, in part because the provider carries an aura of authority and holds a lot of biomedical information.

Similarly, providers likely work more effectively when patients exhibit kindness, trust, and respect. Sometimes patients or their family members treat providers unkindly because they typically do not like the message the provider must deliver about the status of the patient's cancer, because of the limitations on treatment options that the provider can recommend, or because they come from a different cultural background. When comedian Gilda Radner (2009) received a phone call from an oncologist she did not particularly like because he was "gruff and impatient" (p. 206), she berated him, insisted that he reveal the bad news over the phone even though he wanted to talk with her in person, and then argued with him about the blood test results. She knew it was not fair for a patient to punish the provider if you don't like the news that person delivers to you, but she felt justified not only in her reaction but in badgering her physician because she did not feel affiliation in the relationship. This unfair impulse may be a natural reaction to some kinds of information, but it is less likely to occur when the patient and provider have built strong relationship and a history of interpersonal interactions over time.

All providers should consistently exhibit honest communication and reasonable compassion during each interaction, and, though it may be difficult in the unfamiliar and unsettling situation of having cancer, all patients should do the same.

Goal Direction

The third and most important characteristic of provider–patient communication is that it is *goal-directed*, meaning that each interaction is intended to achieve a purpose. Perhaps that goal is to share information about the specifics of a cancer diagnosis, or perhaps that purpose is to decide on specific treatment options for the immediate future. Each interaction should both build the patient–provider relationship and also have goals that address the health situation at hand. Each party—the patient and the provider—may feel responsible for directing goals and must work together as quickly as possible on this aspect of communication.

Here, we adapt the ideas in Erin Meyer's (2014) account of global business interactions in her book *The Culture Map* to help you consider how you judge what is a good meeting with your healthcare provider. "In order for you to feel a meeting was a great success, which of the following should happen?

A. In a good meeting, a decision is made.
B. In a good meeting, various viewpoints are discussed and debated.
C. In a good meeting, a formal stamp is put on a decision that has been made before the meeting." (p. 213)

There is no right or wrong answer. Most Americans tend to choose option A, according to Meyer (2014), whereas most French people choose option B, and most Chinese and Japanese business associates choose option C. Sometimes influenced by one's cultural and social identities in addition to the roles in the specific interaction, the cancer patient frequently measures the success of an interaction with a provider differently than the provider does. When in the cancer care continuum—or for which patients—is it especially beneficial for the provider to enter an interaction with a patient by offering a clear plan of action for the patient to approve? When or for whom is it especially beneficial for the provider to consider various perspectives and debate pros and cons of choices with the patient? How can providers help patients to make their own best decisions? Considering the ways in which decision-making is handled during patient–provider interaction remains an important aspect of cancer care.

Of course, there can be several goals at once for provider–patient communication. Depending on your relationship with your provider and the nature of your illness, your physician may clearly outline the topics for discussion, and you may be able to make clear your needs and expectations for an interaction, too. Often, the provider wants to discuss things the patient wants or needs to know so everyone's goals for the interaction may be in sync without ever being explicitly stated as goals. When a patient does not actively engage in goal-directed communication, physicians and other healthcare providers are likely to assume that their own goals are also the goals of the patient, whether or not that is true. This situation is probably most detrimental to care when a physician and a cancer patient have not discussed potentially divergent goals for both quantity and quality of life.

Sometimes, however, a patient's goals for a visit to the doctor's office or other healthcare facility do not match the goals of the provider. For example, there you are, sitting in a revealing gown on an uncomfortable table under a bright light. Maybe you are nervous, or maybe you have had to wait so long that you drifted off to sleep and feel a bit foggy. Then, the oncologist may walk in reading your chart or jotting notes on a tablet and not make quick eye contact. Despite your right to have undivided attention during a visit with your oncologist, you may find that the provider is distracted by time constraints or by a previous interaction with another patient—maybe this physician just got off the phone with someone like Gilda Radner, who yelled about finding too many cancer markers in her blood. Your physician may rattle off questions because he or she wants to add information to your chart and may not give you cues for more than simple answers. When that is the case, you probably won't feel completely comfortable or successful in your communication with your physician during that visit, even if you thought of several questions in advance, went there with a specific purpose of your own, and tried your best to listen and respond to questions.

These situations can lead to miscommunication or a lack of communication on some topics that are important for the cancer care process. After the patient answers questions and undergoes a physical examination, the physician should turn the conversation over to the patient or invite increased input. "Do you have any questions before I go?" the provider may ask, perhaps genuinely trying to foster interaction. Unfortunately, even if the physician appears relaxed and not rushed, language like *before I go* signals an end soon. In addition, the obvious responses to this call for questions are to either say *no* or to ask a question about the last topic the doctor discussed. As a patient, your best opportunity for shifting the conversation to your questions and goals can easily be missed when it occurs at the end of a visit in which the physician has exerted a lot of control and strong affiliation has not been established.

When the physician exerts control and focuses on predetermined biomedical goals for the interaction, it can be very difficult to get back to other questions or topics that the patient has as goals for the appointment. Questions such as *How will my treatment affect my sexual life?* or *Where can I go to get a good wig?* may seem out of place, perhaps either too difficult to put into words, too complicated to tackle in a few minutes, or too trivial to bother with. If, however, control in the relationship has balanced over time and affiliation is strong, the patient may find it easier to express goals as a patient. Even if it is not so easy, we certainly encourage each patient to work toward your goals in every interaction with healthcare providers. That may mean writing questions down before an appointment, inserting questions into conversations even when it feels a bit awkward, or making a follow-up phone call when the patient is at home, fully dressed, and on familiar turf with pen and paper in hand or web browser open.

Often, patients hope for the best news (or expect the worst news) and, therefore, have not prepared adequate and thoughtful questions, especially when visiting healthcare facilities for routine screenings or early diagnostic tests to confirm suspected cancer. Even after diagnosis, many patients do not prepare questions or bring a friend or family member to appointments, though both tips are touted in many books and brochures about cancer and general health care. When a patient meets with an oncologist, prepared questions can be especially helpful for processing information and making decisions about next steps and long-term health care. Bringing questions can also help patients negotiate control, affiliation, and goal-direction in provider–patient communication for the longer term.

The American Cancer Society recommends versions of the following questions for an initial visit with an oncologist (see "The Doctor-Patient Relationship"). It may be helpful for the patient to bookmark the website on their cell phone or ask the oncologist to look it up to go through the questions important to the patient. Some of these questions may be good to ask in subsequent visits with healthcare providers as well.

- What type of cancer do I have? (This is the diagnosis.)
- What stage is my cancer, and what does that mean? (This is part of the diagnosis, too, and it may be helpful to think about type and stage as separate aspects.)
- What treatment do you recommend for patients with my type and stage of cancer?
- What other treatments can I consider?
- How are these treatments likely to benefit me?
- What are the risks for each treatment?
- How long will it be until you know treatment is working?
- How long will I undergo treatment?
- What side effects, if any, am I likely to experience?
- What can I do to minimize the side effects?

If a patient is not getting clear answers to these types of questions, that individual may want to consider seeking out a different healthcare provider. While switching physicians is not always possible, many patients have options even if they are bound by an insurance plan or a health maintenance organization. Switching healthcare providers is not unusual and should be carefully considered when communication remains an obstacle in cancer care interactions.

Healthcare Provider Training and Practices

Although most nursing schools teach courses in patient–provider communication, it may come as a surprise to patients that physicians receive minimal training in medical school about how to communicate effectively with their patients. Medical school curricula are filled with classes in the sciences, but they do not include many courses on topics such as how to share scientific information in easy-to-understand terms or how to handle emotion or grief during patient interactions. Medical schools and teaching hospitals have recognized the need to include health communication as part of physician training, and, in recent years, many have incorporated simulated patient interactions so that future providers practice basic, well-established principles of health communication.

Because almost every physician has to break bad news to a patient at some point or must guide a patient in decision-making about health care, it is appalling to think that medical students may not practice sharing a cancer diagnosis or convincing a patient who smokes to make specific lifestyle changes. To make up for this lack of in-depth communication education, physicians traditionally do a fair amount of on-the-job learning by trial and error as they begin their medical careers. Often, while the authors of this book advocate formal training in health communication for healthcare providers, strategies for communication are passed down like cultural lore, through observation of elders and idle chatter among peers.

Siddhartha Mukherjee (2010) describes his rigorous on-the-job training in cancer care in his book *The Emperor of All Maladies*. During his fellowship—even after medical school, an internship, and his residency—interacting with real people who had cancer imposed demands on him that he had not expected. He recounts advice from a colleague who had recently finished the two-year fellowship: don't let the immersive training drown you. But Mukherjee

(2010) admits, "The stories of my patients consumed me, and the decisions that I made haunted me" (p. 5). Eventually, he figured out how he could handle communication in ways that worked well for him, including his own spin on the biomedical approach, and for his patients.

Communication policies and habits are also important across the whole cancer care team. In his provocative article "The Checklist," Atul Gawande (2007) points out how agreed-upon checklists for healthcare tasks can seem so simple that they are considered unnecessary but, when used overtly and consistently, lead to better patient care. In addition, Gawande (2007) points out how important it is for nurses to be able—to be authorized formally—to ensure that physicians follow such checklists step by step. While this coordination may seem straightforward to a patient, a hospital culture of strong communication is necessary so that nurses understand that it is their place to remind or question doctors and that such interaction is not confrontation but, rather, represents engaged and coordinated patient care. Gawande (2007) points to studies that show such changes in communication policies and habits—a checklist for the physician, and the nurse double-checking the physician—"were so dramatic that they weren't sure whether to believe them." By the end of a study of patients given a procedure called a central line—a study that lasted well over a year—"the checklist had prevented forty-three infections and eight deaths, and saved two million dollars in costs" (Gawande, 2007).

In other words, communication training and communication practices have a direct bearing on patient outcomes. Checklists and simulations work just as well in health care as they do in aviation, where pilots have used checklists and flight simulators for decades, thereby increasing safety. Open, coordinated communication improves patient care.

The Biomedical Model: Benefits to Patients and Providers

Physicians, including Siddhartha Mukherjee (2010), are usually trained in the *biomedical model* of medicine. This approach to health and illness uses direct evidence and systematic methodology to verify the existence of and treat diseases like cancer. Interactions with providers who adhere very closely to the biomedical approach may be less interactive and more focused on specific, physician-generated questions about symptoms and treatment. Dr. White's approach to his interaction with Kelly Corrigan (2008) exemplifies the strict biomedical approach to communication. According to the biomedical model, communication between providers and patients should be aimed at efficiently sharing information directly relevant to treating the disease.

One positive aspect of the biomedical approach to medicine is that the healthcare provider will put the most emphasis on how to best deal with a patient's cancer. Dealing with the patient's cancer is undoubtedly the top shared priority in provider–patient interactions and across the healthcare team, so this emphasis usually matches patients' overarching goals even when specific goals for a particular conversation may differ. In addition, because time and money are limited resources, the biomedical approach can be advantageous; it narrowly focuses on cancer as a disease that must be addressed in a systematic, efficient manner. Cancer is a physical problem, and the biomedical approach puts the physical nature of the illness front and center in every conversation, every decision, and every test and procedure.

A strictly biomedical approach to provider–patient interactions may be more comfortable for some providers and patients and allow interactions to go more smoothly because the interactions meet expectations even when they do not usually serve everyone's goals. For example, the doctor may say and do what a doctor is likely to say and do, and the patient may respond accordingly with appropriate information, but that does not always mean that the patient leaves the interaction with useful information, greater understanding, or a sense of shared control, affiliation, or goals.

Some physicians and some patients are not comfortable with or adept at talking about difficult personal topics such as the patient's feelings of sadness or anxiety or the impact of the cancer diagnosis on the patient's family, even though these topics also affect the patient's care in various ways. This focus on the physical nature of the disease, without taking into account its personal or cultural implications, tends to keep interactions formal, which, in turn, may be helpful in getting through difficult examinations, complex decisions about treatment, or conversations about a bleak prognosis.

As Mukherjee (2010) suggests, an oncologist can become overwhelmed by the job and use the biomedical approach to maintain some distance and personal equilibrium. Think for a moment about how emotionally difficult it is for healthcare providers to see cancer patients and their families every day. Some patients eventually walk away cancer-free, but some do not survive. A provider who builds a close personal relationship with a patient may feel more responsible for the way that patient's cancer progresses, even though the physician may not be able to control the course of disease. Physicians with close personal relationships with their patients may have trouble feeling they can also be objective about treatment and care options. When patients share a great deal of information with their doctor about their family life, their hopes, and their dreams for life after cancer, the relationship can turn from being purely professional to becoming more of a friendship or partnership in the care process. Though this relationship can sometimes work well, it can be psychologically difficult and emotionally draining for a physician or nurse to manage on a regular basis among many patients. When healthcare providers adhere closely to the biomedical approach, they may be protecting themselves and, ultimately, serving a multitude of patients better in the long run.

Instead of seeking all support from a single provider or facility, a patient may need to seek emotional and spiritual support from other healthcare organizations or outside the traditional healthcare system, perhaps from therapists and counselors, others with cancer, or family and friends. Often, a physician or healthcare organization, a friend with cancer, or a reputable cancer support organization can provide information about additional resources.

Beyond the Biomedical Model

That is certainly not to say that some physicians, physician assistants, nurse practitioners, nurses, or social workers don't develop personal relationships with patients or use informal communication to build a strong partnership as a healthcare team. Nor does this explanation of physician training and communication habits offset the need that many patients have to engage in interactions as an individual with a complex life, a life in which a body with cancer is one part.

Unfortunately, most healthcare clinics and hospitals are not set up to deal with patients as whole people. Instead, they mostly focus on examinations, tests, radiation, chemotherapy, or surgery that address cancer itself. We discuss the role of healthcare organizations and how patients can negotiate these mazes in Chapter 6.

Though physicians have a lot of knowledge about cancer, many are not well skilled at communicating with patients about every aspect of what it means to be a cancer patient. While patients come and go, healthcare providers often spend years in the healthcare setting and, as a result, are comfortable with environments like hospitals and the insider culture that exists there. In contrast, most patients have not spent much time in hospitals or examining rooms and, therefore, are more uncomfortable and anxious in the unfamiliar environment and with a biomedical approach. This difference affects communication and care and should be taken into account by healthcare providers during patient–provider interactions.

While the biomedical approach works well to a great extent, too much reliance strictly on biomedical information sharing can leave out topics that need to be addressed during the cancer care process. Important aspects of the whole person, including one's cultural beliefs, ability to cope with problems, family situation and history, financial status, and even eating habits all play roles in how well that person deals with a cancer diagnosis and responds to treatment. Prognosis may indeed be more than a biomedical question.

In recent years, some healthcare facilities and some physicians have begun to interact more fully with the whole patient. In hospitals, for instance, a patient may have an assigned social worker with whom to discuss the family situation, especially as it relates to caregiving, and the financial situation, especially negotiating paperwork and the costs for the type of care the physician recommends. Some physicians regularly include nutritionists and acupuncturists as part of the healthcare team. As the field of health communication has grown, healthcare facilities and healthcare providers have begun to recognize the need to expand beyond strict adherence to the biomedical model and view each patient as an individual person. As a result, patients are increasingly able to pursue or expect greater whole-person care that benefits them both immediately and in the long run.

Improving Patient–Provider Communication

Statistics Without Stasis and the Role of Emotional Resuscitation

Siddhartha Mukherjee (2010) advocates what he calls *statistics without stasis* as one way to improve patient–provider communication. According to the son who chronicled her illness, Susan Sontag was treated like a child by one physician who meted out the final word on her life and who, perhaps inadvertently, led Sontag to feel hopeless about her situation. She sought out a physician who communicated differently. As Mukherjee (2010) notes:

> Sontag's new physician also told her precisely the same information, without ever choking off the possibility of a miraculous remission. He moved her in succession from standard drugs to experimental drugs to palliative drugs. It was all masterfully done, a graded movement toward reconciliation with death, but a movement nonetheless—statistics without stasis. (p. 307)

Sontag's physician, then, maintained the physician's traditional control in his interactions with her, but he built affiliation and worked to align his goals as a healthcare provider with the goals of his patient for whom options were limited. What may sound misleading or manipulative to some of us may be exactly how a patient needs to hear the information in order to make decisions and live the best life possible. Patients might consider what response they have to this excerpt as a way to gauge how they engage in communication with physicians. Reactions to how Sontag's physician handled her care can reveal important insights for health communication experts.

Same ingredients—same diagnosis, same treatment options, same prognosis—but a different process for putting the information together. Healthcare providers must work to know their patients well enough to adjust the way they convey information so that patients do not become overwhelmed by the amount of information or level of detail or feel compelled to switch messengers. Patients, too, must become aware that a physician may be trying to figure out how best to convey information and decide which information a patient will find most important. Physicians may base the amount of information and the level of detail, for instance, on questions a patient asks. A patient who doesn't ask for information about the stage of one's own cancer or about a prognosis may not be told that information. The lack of a specific request may signal to the physician that the patient is not ready to receive that information yet. Patients can give verbal and body language cues in addition to direct questions, and healthcare providers must look for those cues.

Patients should consider what kind of physicians and interactions they find most useful. In her book *Everybody's Got Something*, television host Robin Roberts (2014), after numerous experiences with the healthcare system, realized, "I had learned from my first battle with cancer that doctors who spout dire statistics don't work for me. I have no doubt that this doctor is a good physician—she came highly recommended. And perhaps there are some patients who find her style refreshing, even reassuring in some way. But it doesn't work for me" (p. 68). Physicians may not be able to adjust their style from patient to patient, and not every patient can switch healthcare providers easily. Those options might be encouraged in some situations, but at the very least, awareness and open communication can help patient and provider work toward shared meaning.

One of Mukherjee's mentors, Thomas Lynch, passed down another strategy for communication that Mukherjee put to use in his own career. According to Mukherjee (2010), Lynch called it *resuscitation*, an approach that "emphasized process over outcome and transmitted astonishing amounts of information with a touch so slight that you might not even feel it" (p. 307). He observed subtle techniques that Lynch used in conversation. Mukherjee (2010) told a patient about the chance of recurrence, for instance, by saying, "Well, there are ways that we will tend to it when that happens" (p. 307). Note the use of *when* not *if*, which orients the patient without scaring her or raising unreasonable expectations. Note the use of *tend* instead of *obliterate*, which lets the patient know that she will receive care but not be cured. Mukherjee compares this sort of cancer communication by a physician to the art of glass blowing, the medical information handled deftly so that it takes a shape that the patient can hold and put to use. Patients, then, must listen carefully not only to what is being said but also to how it is being said and what shape the information is taking.

Whether your cancer is likely curable with relatively standard treatment or whether your cancer is more advanced or difficult to manage, your healthcare providers should help you sort through statistics and other information in ways that help you think about the future as well as the present circumstances. As the Mayo Clinic points out, positive thinking helps a patient deal with stress and even helps the body resist the common cold. While sadness and frustration are appropriate feelings when someone has cancer, we can make choices about our attitudes, and those choices affect our health outcomes and general well-being. Healthcare providers who use honest, thoughtful communication as emotional resuscitation can be especially helpful to patients when the going gets rough in cancer care and can shift conversations in subtle ways to alleviate negative thinking and foster positive attitudes.

Information Avoidance vs. Information Seeking

Let's look more closely at the patient's role in understanding and improving cancer care communication. Basically, there are two approaches by which patients manage communication in the provider–patient interaction: avoiding information or seeking information.

The healthcare provider has information that the patient does not have:

- information about the cancer diagnosis
- information about treatment options
- information about health generally and
- how it applies to the individual patient specifically.

Seeking or avoiding this and other information determines a lot in each interaction the patient has with the healthcare provider.

Some people are *information avoiders*. These patients try to steer clear of sensitive topics and, in doing so, may signal the physician to offer minimal detail or explanation about everything. Information avoiders may engage in small talk with their providers, not as a way to build affiliation but in order to deflect attention from serious topics to trivial matters. Avoiding information can stem from the patient's desire to maintain the identity or role the patient played in society before that person was diagnosed with cancer. As we discuss in Chapter 4, a patient's social identity greatly influences communication and health care. The information avoider may be actively deciding when to tune out information that seems threatening. For instance, that patient may know how cancer is staged generally and that any Stage IV involves metastasis but may not want to know the stage of one's own cancer or may want to delay absorbing that sort of information. This patient may not want to hear or to voice how general information applies to one's own specific situation because that further redefines that person's identity or because the patient needs more time to adjust to the unfamiliar situation.

Information avoiders may be missing important details. Or if you are an information avoider, you may be just as aware as information seekers, though perhaps with less specificity, about the implications of your illness. You also may be trying to filter information and prioritize a small amount of it that matters most to your decisions.

Either way, information avoiders tend to handle their concerns by maintaining privacy, even from their physicians, so that their healthcare providers may be missing important details or making wrong assumptions. Such patients tend to think that having more information will not likely change their attitude or decisions, and some may feel they know themselves well enough that their thoughts and feelings are on point. These patients may not, however, recognize that, in avoiding information themselves, they are keeping valuable information from their healthcare providers. Sometimes, information avoiders inadvertently put their own health at greater risk.

Other people are *information seekers*, or people who enter interactions with a list of questions written down and carefully researched in advance. Information seekers want to know more and often take control of their situations by playing an active role in conversations with their providers. Asking questions, expressing opinions, and voicing concerns are ways that you can become an active participant in your care and feel less powerless over your situation. It is possible that information seekers may be more likely to come across information about clinical trials, experimental drugs, and cutting-edge ideas that may be of use to their care. In addition, active communication and seeking information can help create a strong partnership between the patient and the provider so that, together, they can make decisions about care and solve problems that arise.

Information seekers tend to gather information from a variety of sources and can become overwhelmed or confused, especially when sources contradict each other. A strong partnership with the provider can help the patient filter information collected from the Internet or through friends and family and also apply what is most relevant to the individual situation.

Kelly Corrigan (2008) is an information seeker, not just in response to her own breast cancer diagnosis but even more so in response to her father's bladder cancer diagnosis. She had trouble understanding her parents' reluctance to bother physicians with their questions and her father's resistance to scouring the Internet for every bit of possibly relevant information. While gathering information is usually a positive communication step, gathering every tidbit can create problems. Patients should ask their healthcare providers for a list of trusted websites, and we include several in the appendices of this book.

Corrigan, whose own treatment well very well, inserted herself in her father's care from thousands of miles away, exchanging emails with both her father's physicians to discuss the pros and cons of his treatment options. The physicians didn't agree on the best next step, so Corrigan tried to understand how current cancer care might apply to her father's case. She wanted to take control over the situation, even though she knew, deep down, that she couldn't be in charge of her father's decisions. She criticized herself for the extent to which she wanted to control the flow of information and the decision-making, including the occasional desire for her mother not to play a role in decision-making. Though her father gave her permission to seek information that he was avoiding, decisions about his health care were his to make. While it worked out in their case, she chanced overstepping her role and creating resentment over her interference.

Information seekers often want more information so that they can feel more in control and make better decisions. For many patients, having more information allows them to feel a stronger partnership with their providers and more confident in their cancer care. Information avoiders, on the other hand, may miss opportunities to see all possibilities. Information avoiders like George Corrigan, Kelly's father, sometimes encourage caregivers or family members to seek information on their behalf, allowing the patient to maintain privacy without missing opportunities. Especially without support from others, information avoiders may sometimes put themselves at a disadvantage in interactions and be less informed about the decisions they must make about their care. In the long run, for either an information avoider or an information seeker, a strong relationship with healthcare providers can make a positive difference in decision-making and well-being.

Because information is exchanged in every formal patient–provider interaction, knowing whether you seek or avoid information—or seek some facts while avoiding other details—can help you improve your interactions with your healthcare providers. When healthcare providers develop ongoing relationships with a given patient, they may be better able to communicate with that patient if they know that person's attitude toward information. Ideally, providers will adjust to these different patient approaches without keeping information that may be crucial to decision-making from any patient. A caregiver, too, can play a role in the flow of information and can strengthen communication between the patient and the provider.

Treatment Goals

Some procedures are diagnostic in nature, which means they are designed to give your doctor more information about your cancer. Mammograms and CT scans, for instance, are diagnostic tools. Often, a detailed diagnosis suggests the range—and the limits—for treatment in a specific case. Once the patient and the provider have a clear picture of the illness based on diagnostic tools, they should turn the conversations to the options for the next phase of cancer care. One of the most important topics to discuss with your doctor at this stage of your illness is the goal of your cancer treatment or therapy.

An increasing number of providers are changing the structure of patient interactions to include time before or after an examination for a separate conversation about the situation and next steps. That is one of the best times to talk with your provider about your goals for your care and for your provider to explain the reasonable objectives for each treatment option. Typically, the patient's caregiver or a family member is part of this summary discussion as well. It is easier to take notes during this time than during an examination, which means the patient can keep one's own record of everything that is discussed. In addition, the patient can express individual priorities and ask questions about care in this specific situation. If you have the ability to choose your healthcare providers, you may want to look for those who make these types of separate conversations a routine part of each visit. If you have too few choices about providers and types of interactions, you may want to ask your provider directly how you can get additional information or follow up when you have processed what you have been told.

Depending on the stage of the cancer, the healthcare provider may either offer treatments that seek to cure the cancer, slow the cancer's progress, or manage symptoms the patient experiences as a result of the cancer. In order to make the best choices for oneself, the patient should know which of these three goals the physician sees as reasonable for the specific cancer situation and each treatment option.

Efforts to eradicate the cancer for long-term survival are therapies that healthcare providers use in a *curative approach* to fighting disease. Such therapies are usually designed to cure cancer that is still in its early stages and has not spread when the diagnosis is made. The primary goal of curative surgeries, curative radiation therapies, curative immunotherapy, or other curative treatments is to remove or destroy all cancer cells. Often physicians do not like to use the term *cure* because they cannot predict the outcome of treatment or whether the cancer will recur. Physicians may refer to a person as being *cancer free* instead of being cured.

Curative treatments are not reasonable options for all stages of cancer, and not all surgery, radiation, chemotherapy, or immunotherapy is designed to be curative. Though a patient may be afraid of the answer, an individual may want to ask bluntly whether it is reasonable to expect to be cancer free in the future. That information is likely to affect a range of decisions about cancer care. If the physician indicates that your cancer is eminently curable, you may want to consider your own priorities before you ask for more information, including the chances for cure in statistical terms.

Would it change your decision to pursue a particular treatment option, for instance, if that treatment had a 20% chance of cure instead of a 90% chance? Would you pursue a long-shot cure at age 50 that you would not pursue at 75 years of age? These hypothetical questions become more complex when a patient must decide between several treatment options, each of which has different chance of working—what is called efficacy—and risk associated with it. Having an honest conversation about realistic outcomes helps minimize misunderstandings between patient and providers and helps the patient make the best decision about the next steps in care.

Robin Roberts (2014) recounts in her book *Everybody's Got Something* that, after grueling chemotherapy treatment for breast cancer, she would never go through anything like that again. But when she was diagnosed with MDS, a precursor to cancer if it were not aggressively treated, she changed her mind. Why? The possibility of a cure changed her decision about whether to undergo aggressive treatment.

Astoundingly, some patients do not acquire enough useful information for fully informed decision-making and, therefore, undergo treatment without a strong understanding of how the intended goal of treatment matches their individual goals. In some ways, this situation is understandable and sometimes stems from basic miscommunication. No one wants to hear bad news, and medical terminology and language usage may be unfamiliar. Positive thinking is important, but not at the expense of relevant information and situation-appropriate understanding.

An information seeker may have gathered conflicting information about surgery or may not have sorted through how different versions of a surgical procedure apply to different stages of a particular type of cancer, for instance. Or an information avoider who has not directly asked whether the cancer has spread may not understand that surgery might be used either to cure early-stage cancer or to extend life for a few months in more advanced cancer. In other words, not all surgery—or any other treatment—has the same goal in every situation, but without a clear explanation about the specific circumstances, a patient may assume that surgery is not going to be done unless it is going to eradicate cancer.

On the flip side, patients sorting through unfamiliar medical terminology coming out of an oncologist's mouth may feel overwhelmed. The words may seem ominous, when the physician is actually conveying an optimistic prognosis or treatment objectives. Sometimes, neither patient nor provider realize miscommunication has occurred until later, perhaps after next steps in cancer care have already been taken.

Former astronaut Sally Ride had extensive surgery for pancreatic cancer. However, during surgery, her physicians discovered that, though the disease had not yet spread to other organs, the cancer was more extensive than the diagnostic tools had indicated. A few months after surgery, Ride's health was still declining, so she underwent chemotherapy and radiation therapy in hopes of improving. She had made the initial decision to undergo aggressive treatment, according to Lynn Sherr's (2014) book, because she expected to get better. Often, one treatment leads to another, sometimes without much discussion between provider and patient about how new information or changing circumstances affect future options and decisions. When her healthcare providers brought up hospice less than a year after surgery, Ride was taken by surprise.

As we saw at the beginning of this chapter with Kelly Corrigan's experience being diagnosed with breast cancer, a physician may focus on the next step, and a patient may not have several potential future scenarios in her head. Though she was incredibly well educated, Ride may not have fully understood what the surgery had revealed and what that result meant for her long-term prognosis. According to her physician, when Ride was faced with the suggestion of hospice, she adjusted quickly, maintained her positive attitude, and asked whether the progress of the disease could be slowed. Slowing the progress of pancreatic cancer is often an objective for therapies because that cancer is usually diagnosed at a later stage of development, so Ride's options probably had been narrowing toward hospice for a while. She had a can-do personality, preferring to know what could be done, and then she dealt with each situation as it presented itself.

To avoid miscommunication or false expectations about the potential benefits and harms that might come from a particular therapy or procedure, communication with your provider is the only solution. While most people would agree it is beneficial to use available medications and procedures to save a person from suffering, the nature of cancer can make this a complicated issue for the individual patient. If surgery will cure your cancer and you are in otherwise good health, you are likely to want to undergo surgery. But what if your surgery is not curative? What will you do if surgery will extend your life by only several months and if the recovery from that surgery will be physically difficult in addition to having cancer itself? What if you have other health conditions that increase the risk of surgery? Or you may be faced with a decision that involves multiple components or possible combinations, such as surgery, chemotherapy, and radiation. Some patients may want to try every possible treatment, whereas others may not.

Given the variety of scenarios, it is important to remember that cancer care decisions for similar or equal conditions of a diagnosis and related prognosis can vary greatly from family to family and are often influenced by one's host culture and/or cultural background. Some patients will find decisions that negotiate quality and quantity of life to be more straightforward than other patients. Decision-making around cancer care and treatment is a very personal decision that can sometimes seem peculiar to others, especially those outside the family. For instance, patients and families from collectivistic cultures often want to save face—maintain respect and avoid embarrassment—for their loved ones during the cancer journey. This can play out in a number of ways when it comes to decisions about moving forward with treatments. By undergoing aggressive treatment, the patient can show the family the patient is trying everything to live as long as possible despite a dire diagnosis and prognosis. In turn, the family often may engage in similar saving face behaviors such as deciding to not turn to hospice care, as that could be perceived as giving up on their loved one in the fight to live longer. Other patients or families who are faced with a dire diagnosis and prognosis may slowly—or sometimes quickly—shift their focus from seeking aggressive treatment to discussing end-of-life or even afterlife.

Honest dialogue is often necessary for a patient to express one's priorities so that the physician can make appropriate and reasonable recommendations—and adjust goals—for cancer care. When that happens, providers can help their patients maintain a positive and realistic—informed—attitude that cultivates the best life possible during cancer care and for the future.

Risks, Side Effects, and Double Binds

Some patients handle some forms of chemotherapy with few side effects. Depending on the treatment, the patient may never miss a day of work. When talking with the physician about different approaches, however, the patient should encourage an honest conversation about negative implications for quality of life, from nausea, neuropathy, and hair loss as a result of chemotherapy to fatigue and muscle weakness from radiation treatment to time spent in the hospital or a rehabilitation center while recovering from surgery to the risk of infection from any of these treatment options.

In addition to the objectives of each treatment, the conversation between the patient and the provider should address side effects and risks for each treatment option. Chemotherapy, radiation, immunotherapy, and other treatments may fight the disease only temporarily, and sometimes—depending on the cancer and its stage, the specific treatment regimen, and the patient's overall health—the side effects are difficult to bear. Such treatments should not necessarily be dismissed but, rather, discussed in the context of the specific situation and options for managing side effects and risks.

Susan Gubar (2012), in her book *Memoir of a Debulked Woman*, chronicles her treatment for ovarian cancer. Ovarian cancer is very curable when it is detected early, but it is often detected at later stages and, therefore, according to the American Cancer Society, has an overall five-year survival rate of less than 50%. Gubar (2012) admits, "Only months after the diagnosis did I finally understand the prognosis established at the debulking [surgery]. Had Dr. Stehman refrained from going into details that might be discouraging or was his language simply incomprehensible to me?" (p. 241) She found herself, as do many patients with advanced cancer, in a double-bind months after surgery. Gubar ended up with an abscess and perforation as a result of the debulking surgery—something that was a surprise to her but not to her physicians. She was then faced with choosing between a relatively minor repair surgery with a low chance of success and a major surgery with a higher chance of success but also a higher risk of death. Because cancer treatment options carry significant risks and sometimes have severe side effects, Gubar's experience is not unusual for patients with advanced stages of cancer (i.e., stage III or IV).

Gilda Radner (2009) also was treated for ovarian cancer. Though her treatment occurred in the 1980s, and cancer care has changed since then in many ways, her account of side effects from chemotherapy and a kind of double bind remain relevant for some patients.

> The numbness had increased a lot in my arms and legs. My legs, which had been numb below the knee, were now numb above the knee into the thigh. I had noticed it, but I had gotten used to it. When I walked on my feet it felt like I had on huge boots filled with sand. My arms were numb almost to the shoulder. I could still play tennis, but when I would feel in my pockets, I couldn't distinguish between objects. (p. 189)

The neuropathy had become so bad that her gynecological oncologist worried that this side effect would become worse with the next chemotherapy treatment and possibly permanently disabling. Cutting chemotherapy short meant a lower chance of eliminating all microscopic cancer cells, but continuing chemotherapy meant a greater chance of severe physical disability. Her physician recommended starting a full round—thirty daily treatments—of radiation therapy instead, even though it was less effective and had its own set of side effects.

Syncing Treatment Goals with Individual Goals

While physicians often cannot predict which side effects or risks are most likely for an individual patient, understanding the possibilities that pertain to you and your cancer can help you make choices. In early-stage cancer, especially in a young and otherwise healthy patient, the decisions about treatment may be relatively simple to make because the benefits are great and the risks are low. Some patients with advanced cancer may choose aggressive treatments that result in feeling sick and losing hair in order to have more time with family and friends. Other patients whose cancer cannot be cured may choose palliative medication to alleviate pain in order to feel better during remaining time with family and friends, even if that means less time with loved ones. Understanding the range of possibilities, especially when there is no ideal choice, no obviously good or bad option, is an important goal for provider–patient communication.

Physicians must recognize that no cancer treatment option is a one-size-fits-all, and patients must take an active role in deciding their treatment. Eve Ensler wrote, "I am a you-will-not-destroy-me-as-you're-whipping-me person. I am an I-will-find-a-way-out-of-this person. We all do what we do to survive. Cynicism. Optimism. Both paths require work" (p. 184). To make the best decisions for oneself, patients might consider whether they are cynics or optimists and also whether they value quantity or quality of life more. Of course, most of us are cynical sometimes and optimistic at other times. Most of us would like to have both quantity (more time) and quality (greater satisfaction or enjoyment) in our lives. When cancer interferes with achieving the goals you had for your life before the diagnosis, you may need to negotiate or compromise in order to make the best life possible for yourself. How can you and your healthcare providers best sync up your goals in life with the options your physician recommends based on his or her goals for cancer care? What are your priorities in life? And how can you make decisions that reflect and cultivate those priorities?

Exercise & Discussion

This role-playing scenario allows students to work in pairs (one person as healthcare provider, the other as patient) to explore provider–patient interactions, including how patients respond to providers, how providers respond to patients, and how patients respond to caregivers. We offer suggestions to get started, and participants can create their own scenarios.

Consider the distinct and shared goals of each person in the exchange. Also, consider how to build shared meaning even if the goals of the patient and the provider are not all shared. Keep in mind how socialized into the healthcare organization the patient is when the exchange occurs. You can refer to the website of the American Cancer Society, the National Cancer Institute, or another organization for information you can use in these exchanges.

SCENARIO 1
Radiologist: Your MRI shows a mass. When you leave today, you can schedule a biopsy.
Patient: ____

SCENARIO 2
Oncologist: The biopsy indicates pre-cancerous cells.
Patient: ____

SCENARIO 3
Patient: Am I going to die from this?
Oncologist: ____

SCENARIO 4
Patient: How will I feel during chemo treatment?
Oncologist: ____

SCENARIO 5
Caregiver: I'm worried that you're dehydrated. Should we go to the ER?
Patient: ____

Now, construct your own possible provider–patient interactions.

References

Corrigan, K. (2008). *The middle place*. New York, NY: Hyperion.

Ensler, E. (2013). *In the body of the world*. New York, NY: Metropolitan.

Gawande, A. (2007). The checklist. *The New Yorker* December 10, 2007. Retrieved from http://www.newyorker.com/magazine/2007/12/10/the-checklist

Gubar, S. (2012). *Memoir of a debulked woman*. New York, NY: W.W. Norton.

Huntington, B., & Kuhn, N. (2003). Communication gaffes: A root cause of malpractice claims. *Baylor University Medical Center Proceedings*, *16*, 157–161.

Levinson, W., Roter, D., Mullooly, J., Dull, V. & Frankel, R. Physician–patient communication: The relationship with malpractice claims among primary care physicians and surgeons. *Journal of the American Medical Association*, *277(7)*, 553–559. doi: 10.1001/jama.1997.03540310051034

Meyer, E. (2014). *The culture map: Breaking through the invisible boundaries of global business*. New York, NY: Public Affairs.

Mukherjee, S. (2010). *The emperor of all maladies*. New York, NY: Scribner.

Radner, G. (1989/2009). *It's always something*. New York, NY: Simon & Schuster.

Roberts, R. (2014). *Everybody's got something*. New York, NY: Grand Central.

Sherr, Lynn (2014). *Sally Ride: America's first woman in space*. New York: Simon & Schuster.

Sparks, L., & Villagran, M. (2010). *Patient and provider interaction: A global health communication perspective*. Cambridge: Polity Press.

Wright, K. B., Sparks, L., & O'Hair, H. D. (2013). *Health communication in the 21st century* (2nd ed.). Oxford: Blackwell.

·8·

GIVING CARE, TAKING CARE

Caregivers and Communication

the clock is moving and not moving
the monitor is beeping and not beeping
the nurse is coming and not coming

time is passing and not passing

my mother is seeing and not seeing
my mother is hearing and not hearing
my mother is breathing and not breathing

I am seeing her face and not seeing her face
I am hearing her voice and not hearing her voice
I am squeezing her hand and not squeezing her hand

I am beside her and beside myself

—from "In the ICU" by Lesléa Newman

When Lisa Sparks's father John Otho Sparks, a long-time smoker, was diagnosed with cancer, it had already spread beyond his lungs. At 57 years of age, he was facing Stage IV cancer with 16 metastatic lesions on his brain. Lisa was finishing her graduate-school work at the University of Oklahoma, near where her father lived. Working on her doctoral dissertation had seemed like the most important focus for her life until her father became ill. Though she was not her father's primary caregiver, she played an important role as a secondary caregiver. There was no chance for a cure in his case, but he underwent aggressive chemotherapy to extend his life. Lisa thinks that part of the reason he made this decision was to have the chance to see his first grandchild, Elena. Between the progression of the disease and the side effects of the treatment, he needed to be taken to many medical appointments and also required at-home care as his abilities deteriorated. Lisa helped with those tasks, sometimes doing laundry in the middle of the night at the hospital and changing her father's clothing, often feeling as if the parent and child roles had been reversed, which, she knew, must have been especially hard on her father.

Years later, despite the grief she still feels over losing her father at a young age, Lisa remains grateful that, when her father needed caregiving during the last year of his life, she was at a point in her life when she could adjust her schedule and obligations to spend a significant amount of time with him. Much research in health communication focuses on provider–patient interaction. As the authors know from their own experiences as caregivers in addition to their work as scholars, caregiver–patient interaction is an important component of cancer communication.

Roles of the Caregiver

While healthcare providers offer medical care, a cancer diagnosis often leads to the need for other kinds of caregiving like that Lisa offered for her father. Sometimes, a cancer diagnosis may mean numerous family members and friends pitching in to help with various tasks, but sometimes family members will thrust themselves into—or be thrust into—the role of primary caregiver for a parent with cancer. As Lee Brock, Lisa's cousin (the sister she never had), said when she talked with the authors about the different roles she and her brothers took in caring for their mother (Lisa's aunt, Sue Brock) with cancer, "Sometimes people can only do what they can do so they do what they can do." It is important but not easy for a family to figure out who can do what as caregivers.

Both formal and informal social networks are often involved in the cancer care process. Formal caregivers include the various healthcare providers a patient will encounter from the time of a cancer diagnosis through treatment, including the primary care physician, oncologist, nurses, nursing aides, and various technologists. Formal caregivers like nurses offer care because it is their job, and they are recognized by the culture as trained caregivers. *Informal caregivers* typically include family members and close friends but also can include other people involved in the patient's care who are outside the formal healthcare system, including a minister or even a hairdresser. Successful negotiation of the various intersections and interactions between formal and informal caregiving is called *balanced coordination*. This balanced coordination of all the different caregivers and kinds of care is extremely important after a cancer diagnosis. Balanced coordination among the various formal and informal caregivers can be tricky, especially because vast amounts of health information must be sorted through and deciphered, sometimes piecemeal by different caregivers, so that the best decisions can be made for each patient and cancer situation.

Some of the many responsibilities with which an informal caregiver or group of caregivers might contend include the following:

- providing physical assistance to the patient, including following instructions about medical care from healthcare providers;
- serving as a liaison between the patient and the team of healthcare providers, including monitoring symptoms and communicating them to providers;
- providing emotional support to the patient;
- handling financial affairs for the patient, perhaps including holding Power of Attorney for financial decision making and account access; and
- handling social affairs and personal correspondence, which may include phone calls and email, for the patient.

Though we think of *care* as meaning *help or assistance*, the Old English meaning of the word is *sorrow, anxiety, or grief*. When someone outside the formal healthcare system offers to care for a cancer patient, it often emerges out of a generous form of sorrow, as well as a genuine desire to help a loved one. But caregiving can be a response to anxiety, too, over the diagnosis and what it means for the patient and the family. Though this anxiety in no way diminishes the generosity or the effort, sometimes people offer care to alleviate their own anxiety and address their own need to do something active to try to make the situation better.

As the physical and emotional responsibilities go on, caregiving itself can cause anxiety for the person offering care. *Care* has another meaning as well:

serious mental attention. This attention is necessary in caregivers but can be exhausting, especially because the progression of a specific cancer, treatment timelines, and effects of treatment are unpredictable for a given patient.

Professional caregivers can be a helpful part of the caregiving team. Relatively few people in our society, however, have the financial means to afford a professional caregiver for their loved ones, so they take on the responsibility themselves. In fact, S. Lochlann Jain (2013) mentions, in her book about cancer, that 46 percent of cancer patients receive calls from collection agencies, and some experts attribute the majority of personal bankruptcies to the cost of catastrophic illness. Financial burdens of cancer care can cause stress for the patient and the patient's family, and cost can be a determining factor in managing caregiving. Patients should be honest with their healthcare providers so that those providers know what options and limitations in caregiving might affect medical care and treatment efficacy and so that patients, providers, and caregivers can coordinate the best possibilities for care that is needed.

When they become caregivers, spouses, life partners, and other family members may spend an enormous amount of time and energy meeting the physical needs of a patient. But most people do not have the experience, skills, or training to handle the immense physical and cognitive responsibility of caregiving with ease. Health literacy and health communication, which we discussed earlier, are important issues for caregivers, but additional aspects of this vital role need to be considered as well.

Communication skills are crucial for caregivers, both in serving the needs of the patient and in making sure that their own needs don't get lost in the shuffle of roles. *Communication competence* refers to an individual's capacity to form and implement context-appropriate and effective messages that also meet the goals or needs of the participants. This competence in the communicative act is part of what allows a person to make and sustain satisfying relationships over time. Not everyone achieves high communication competence in every situation, but it is an especially important characteristic to consider when thinking about informal caregivers. Researchers, for instance, have found that caregivers with higher communication competence created relationships in which older adults with cancer reported lower stress levels and higher satisfaction with their support networks than individuals who had caregivers with lower communication competence (Bevan & Sparks, 2011). Communicating well makes the unwanted situation of cancer easier for everyone involved to manage.

Caregiving and Gender

We wrote about gender in Chapter 3 and Chapter 4, where we discuss in depth how culture and social identity affect cancer care. While we focused there especially on the patient and the patient's interactions with physicians, gender is an important factor in informal caregiving as well. Informal caregiving is often established without much discussion, and being the child of someone with cancer or being the spouse of someone with cancer puts you in the most likely positions for caregiving. While decisions often emerge from these existing relationships, a caregiver may fall into the role quickly without knowing what it really entails. Being aware of factors such as gender will help both patients and caregivers talk about the options for caregiving, how to adapt existing roles and relationships to the new situation, and make the best decisions possible for their situations.

In most societies in the 21st century, women are much more likely than men to become caregivers. That is what happened when Lee Brock's mother (Lisa's aunt, Sue Brock) was diagnosed with cancer. Though Lee had two brothers, she bore the heaviest responsibility for caring for her mom. Lee went to all of her mother's medical appointments after the diagnosis and regularly visited her mother, who lived alone, especially to bring healthy nutritional foods including protein shakes. For stretches, Lee visited her mother every day, sometimes twice a day, though her mother often shooed Lee away after twenty minutes. Lee's mother needed the caregiving but also wanted to remain as self-sufficient as possible. When she could barely get her mother to a doctor's appointment, Lee was the one to begin inquiring about hospice services and, during a downturn, needed to quickly get her mother to the hospital for the scan that revealed that the cancer had spread throughout the body. Together, Lee and her mother decided when to bring the brothers home for some time with their mother. In the final days, her mother received medical care in the hospital, and Lee welcomed her brothers and her cousin, Lisa Sparks (one of this book's authors). At that point, she saw her role with her mother as "shepherding her into the next phase." Lisa helped to subtly guide the family through the most difficult end-of-life phase as she witnessed many communicative cues from the healthcare team that indicated transitions to death. Some people are more attuned to such communicative cues than others due to differences in experiences with the disease, hospital systems, and emotional and cognitive processing abilities during times of crisis, as well as with family dynamics that emerge in unique ways during such uncertain times.

The Family Caregiver Alliance (2003) pulled together a variety of information in its report "Women and Caregiving: Facts and Figures." Importantly, most informal caregivers are women, and female caregivers devote significantly more time to caregiving than do male caregivers. Many women caregivers, according to this report, are married and employed, and many incur significant financial strain related to their caregiving. That is not to say that men aren't good caregivers nor that they don't step into the role. These cultural contexts and assumptions tend to influence caregiving, whether the caregiver is male or female.

Because women are often stereotyped as more nurturing than men and because men are stereotyped as breadwinners, women are sometimes assumed to be better suited as caregivers and in a better position to adjust their lives—including their work schedules—to accommodate caregiving than are men. A recent study called "When Gender Trumps Everything: The Division of Parent Care Among Siblings" (Grigoryeva, 2014) found that daughters spend twice as much time caring for elderly parents as do sons, that sons are less likely to take on care if daughters are available, and that daughters will put in extra caregiving time to compensate when sons slack off. Unfortunately, these cultural conditions and expectations have led to a situation in which women have had to bear the brunt of caregiver responsibilities in many societies, and men serve as back-up caregivers. In addition, in the United States, many female caregivers are older themselves, sometimes living on fixed incomes, with limited financial resources, or limited social resources (Sparks, 2013).

The Family Communication Patterns model offers one way to understand caregiving and other health issues within families. This model categorizes families as consensual, pluralistic, protective, or laissez-faire in order to understand communication patterns within families. A recent study used this model as the basis for interviews with eight Australian mother–daughter dyads to analyze the potential for daughters to communicate information—convey health information messages—about screening mammography to their mothers. The results were consistent with those of previous studies conducted in other cultural contexts and indicated reciprocal relationships between mothers and daughters in which the Australian mother–daughter dyads frequently communicated about health topics. In addition, daughters were a source of health information and influenced their mothers' decision-making about mammography. The delivery from daughter to mother of mammography promotion messages may be most successful for dyads and cultures that highly value reciprocal conversations (Browne, & Chan, 2012).

A spouse of someone with cancer—whether male or female, whether middle-aged or elderly—is often positioned well in relation to the patient for the bulk of caregiving responsibilities. Spousal caregivers often provide more wide-ranging care over longer periods of time than do other informal caregivers (Sparks, 2013). That makes sense. Couples who share a household tend to be *there* already for caregiving. But caregiving often entails a variety of tasks and also often requires adjustments to life beyond the home, including adjusting work hours.

Numerous studies of couples dealing with cancer indicate that the spouse is the most important source of emotional support and that emotional support has a big impact on how a person copes with a serious illness (Bevan & Sparks, 2011; Sparks, 2013). Couples should be aware that a cancer diagnosis and the ensuing need for caregiving tend to heighten whatever kind of relationship the couple had before the diagnosis. Marital tension that existed before the diagnosis is likely to be exacerbated by a cancer diagnosis and caregiving. On the other hand, a strong relationship that shifts into patient–caregiver mode can often increase the closeness the couple feels and improve communication (Sparks, 2013).

Research indicates that, when men are thrust into caregiving for their wives, the men sometimes struggle to adopt what are likely several new, gender-switching roles for them. Many men tend not to think of themselves as good at household tasks, for instance, or at personal care. Even women who work outside the home, on the other hand, tend to do more housework and merely extend those existing roles when caregiving becomes part of their lives. Male caregivers may become overwhelmed by unfamiliar tasks at home and seek additional helpers for household chores, and their wives may worsen the situation by pointing out shortcomings (Bevan, Vreeburg, Verdugo, & Sparks, 2012).

Talking openly about priorities—how important is it to fold the laundry properly? what should be done today and what can wait?—and recognizing that it's difficult for one person to fill another's shoes can help the spousal patient and caregiver establish new ways of working together. Though much less research exists about caregiving in same-sex couples (Kamen et al., 2015), this honest discussion about priorities is likely useful no matter the gender of the patient or caregiver, whether the couple is same or opposite sex, and regardless of whether either partner fits stereotypical roles.

In addition, talking about shared concerns, such as fear of cancer recurrence, is an important part of partnered caregiving. It is easy to think of the patient's concerns as only the patient's concerns, but spouses often share the same concerns and, in a way, live with cancer every day as well (Sparks, 2013). Individuals often deal with shared concerns differently, and some of those differences in approach are related to social identity. For partners who are caregivers, worry about the future and other daily stresses can cause sleep disruption, eating disorders, depression, and grief. Men often have greater difficulty adjusting to the demands of caregiving and higher rates of such symptoms of distress. In a three-year study of spousal caregivers, husbands' psychological state tended to worsen steadily, whereas wives showed less distress over time and greater ability to adjust (Bevan & Sparks, 2011; Sparks, 2013).

Part of this difference in coping might be attributed to gendered communication styles, with men less likely to talk about their concerns and anxiety because they don't want to appear weak to themselves or others (Bevan & Sparks, 2011). Especially for male caregivers, talking openly may be important to maintaining attentive caregiving over time and preserving the strength of existing relationships. In addition, finding ways to take action—gather information, participate in doctor visits, administer medications—is likely to help men adjust more quickly and deeply to caregiving roles (see Sparks, 2013).

Caregiving shared across genders offers a more flexible, fluid informal caregiver system for society and individuals. Hopefully, in the future, as societal ideas about gender and marriage continue to shift, increases in shared caregiving responsibilities across and within families will give patients more options and greater support. Even today, honest, inclusive discussions within families can help to create a plan for caring for a loved one with cancer or an aging family member.

Few people want to face the most basic fact of every life: that it will end. End-of-life fears, priorities, and decisions can be difficult for the patient, family and caregivers, and even healthcare providers to face. For some individuals, talking about these issues while healthy makes the conversations easier, and we recommend that any adult consider these questions before a cancer diagnosis. In addition to talking with healthcare providers and spiritual counselors, a patient may want to talk with a lawyer or with a friend who has dealt with the death of a close family member or to search the Internet for answers to some of the following questions, knowing that laws and practices vary from country to country and from state to state.

- If I were incapacitated, who would make my healthcare decisions? How can I designate a specific person to do that? If I don't designate someone, who makes my healthcare decisions if I am not able to do so?
- What is the difference between a *living will* and a *power of attorney*? How can I have one or both documents so that my priorities are considered even if I am not able to make healthcare decisions myself?
- Should I consider a separate power of attorney for health care and for finances? If someone is not designated to take care of my finances for me, how do my bills get paid?
- What is a DNR, or do-not-resuscitate, order? Can I change my mind after I have signed a DNR? How do healthcare professionals who might treat me know whether I have signed a DNR?
- Who decides what happens to my remains? If someone else makes arrangements for my cremation or burial, how do they know what I want?
- Do I need a *probate attorney* to help get my affairs in order? What is the difference between a *probate attorney* and a general *attorney or lawyer*?
- How can I write or update a will? Who should be the executor? What happens to my assets and belongings if I die without a will?

Caregiving Affects the Whole Family

Research has shown, again and again, that the serious illness of one member of a family affects the lives of not only the patient but also the family and loved ones. Because of these findings, several scholars assert that a serious illness is an issue for the entire family (Sparks, 2003, 2013). A cancer diagnosis adds new demands to families, as emotional strains and financial hardships may increase and as the increased mental attention to caregiving reorients day-to-day life for everyone in the family. Numerous changes in routine as well as treatment schedules and other decisions affect the entire family, and families may perform caregiving without even thinking of it by that term. A patient and that person's family may feel disoriented by a new way of life and interactions with the unfamiliar places, people, and language of formal cancer care.

Add to this the likelihood that not everyone in the family will agree on all aspects of care, heightening tension within the family. Lee Brock faced such situations with her mother, Sue Brock. Her mother was not always an acquiescent patient. Though she gave up smoking and drinking for surgery, after surgery, she would turn her oxygen off to smoke. She sometimes canceled follow-up care appointments, which made it more difficult for Lee to offer consistent care and more difficult for her mother to remain as able to care for herself or move around. They sometimes disagreed about when to inform the brothers about information, so Lee, in the end, followed her mother's cues on family communication. For a family caregiver, it can be especially complicated to negotiate issues of control and decision-making.

A pioneering study on the prioritizing of family communication used the theory of socioemotional selectivity to look at the effects of kinship on women's health and aging. Fisher and Nussbaum (2015) found that an individual's choice of partner and ongoing interpersonal communication play a fundamental role in overall well-being, are oriented for survival and goals related to survival, and play a role in optimizing health. In fact, interpersonal communication within families is especially important to wellness over a lifespan. Effective and loving communication among family members helps each individual adapt to stress, cope, and adapt to aging (Fisher & Nussbaum, 2015).

Therefore, despite these demands, families are often uniquely qualified to understand patient attitudes and decision-making strategies and can assist as an important resource in helping the patient to make better decisions about care. Most older adults in the United States who are dependent on others and who require long-term care currently receive that care from members of their own families. In turn, many of those caregivers are middle-aged adults thrust into that caregiving role for their older family members while still caring for their own children as well (Sparks, 2013). Such family caregivers are termed *The Sandwich Generation* due to the competing roles of caring for older and younger members of the family.

Perhaps, the most important element the new caregivers must remember is to first take care of themselves. A stable, healthy, positive caregiver can truly have more to offer to the family member with cancer. Caregivers must continue to take some time out for themselves so they can be there when the patient needs them throughout the various phases of the cancer care process.

Stressed Out: The Demands of Caregiving

Caregiving is an extremely difficult and stressful job, and, in most cases when family members or friends offer care, it is unpaid labor. Caring for a family member over the continuum of cancer care can be an emotionally and physically demanding experience for the caregiver. Dealing with cancer often becomes a fulltime job—or at least a fulltime mental and physical attitude—for the patient and can also become a fulltime job for the primary informal caregiver. The patient and the caregiver both face the influx of doctor appointments, medical tests, chemotherapy and radiation regimens, and other tasks on what often becomes a mutual or shared schedule. In addition, caregivers sometimes may expend significant effort hiding their emotions and concerns from the patient in an effort to minimize the burdens the patient may feel along the care journey.

When the diagnosis is made and a treatment plan is laid out and agreed upon between the patient and the provider, the caregiver may have a sense of how long caregiving will be needed. But a physician may not account for unexpected circumstances, like a delayed chemotherapy treatment because of a low white blood cell count or because of an infection that requires additional treatment with antibiotics. Also, the physician may not talk about the long-term care needs beyond the next phase of treatment, instead wanting the patient to take things step by step, making decisions along the way. Lee Brock, in our interview with her, definitely felt as if she became very focused on task after task and had trouble keeping the big picture in mind, perhaps even using a task as a kind of denial about anything beyond that moment. In other words, when a family member commits to caregiving, that person may not fully realize the extent to which the actual caregiving itself will make demands.

When Carla Malden's (2011) husband was diagnosed with colorectal cancer, she tried to absorb information during his appointments and prepare herself for the caregiving role into which she'd been thrust. In *Afterimage*, she writes:

> The nurse handed us drug company pamphlets and a royal-blue tote bag. Inside were fleece gloves intended to bring relief from the neuropathy threatened by the Oxaliplatin. I had no idea what that meant. Neuropathy. She explained the condition—numbness, tingling, iciness of the extremities—but we didn't really understand the potential severity. How bad could it be if a pair of plush gloves in this lovely swag bag could make it better? She cautioned Laurence against reaching into the refrigerator and to avoid icy drinks, warning that the nerve damage could become permanent. Still, I thought, *No nerve damage for us. We're on our way back to normal.* (p. 65)

Chemotherapy was not just something that Laurence would go into the healthcare facility to receive; it was something that would determine caregiving at home to a great extent. But when she was first taking in all the information, Carla Malden minimized, in her thoughts, the effects it would have on the lives of her husband and herself.

While her positive attitude helped the couple cope, experience changed her outlook. She had not expected cancer to change Laurence mentally and emotionally as well as physically. Sometimes, those changes in him increased her anxiety dramatically. For her, as his wife and his primary caregiver, she had to adapt to these unexpected circumstances. When she read about chemotherapy side effects or about the stress of caregiving, she did not want to think it could happen to her. "Despite various books people offered on caregiving," Malden (2011) wrote, "all of which discussed the caregiver's inevitable resentment toward the patient, the fury only split me further. I was angry and I was guilty and I was ashamed. I was out of control" (p. 138).

An offer of or need for caregiving often emerges quickly from an immediate situation—a cancer diagnosis, a treatment schedule—but caregiving can be a long-term commitment. The caregiver must remain strong and steady for the months and perhaps years of a caregiving marathon. In order to be ready for a marathon, a runner takes time to run and exercise every day. The runner must put in proper mileage each week in order to be prepared for the marathon that is scheduled a few months away. A proper diet must be followed, and sleep becomes a top priority as race day approaches. Running with a partner is often helpful social support that aids in accomplishing milestones that lead to the marathon. Just like a marathon runner, the caregiver must take time to train for the caregiving journey that lies ahead. The runner may measure the effort in miles, and the caregiver also measures effort by the amount of emotional and physical energy expended.

Robin Romm (2009) wrote about her experience as one of her mother's primary caregivers during the final weeks when her mother was in home hospice care with cancer:

> I have refused to do night shifts with my mother. I can tell that everyone is trying hard not to judge me, but I know my limits, and I am already so far past them that a night alone on duty at this point, when nights and days have stopped meaning anything to my mother and she's frequently up every single hour of every day, will ruin me. (p. 146)

Romm understood that pushing herself beyond her limits risked her ability to stick with the caregiving over time and do it as well as she could for as long as she was needed. Romm was able to take into account her limits because she shared caregiving with her father and, to a lesser extent, with a few family friends as well as with the hospice nurses who stopped by to check on the situation.

Amber, the partner and caregiver for television host Robin Roberts (2014), faced a similar situation and, in hindsight, would recommend to other caregivers that they take time for themselves. Even if the patient and caregiver have relocated for treatment, Amber urges caregivers to seek out a gym, yoga studio, or some place to clear your mind and recharge physically. That is the only way to keep going over time.

Often, the social support needs for the caregiver are as important as for the cancer patient. For a caregiver as well as for a patient, this is a journey like none experienced or imagined before. The cancer patient and family members go through stages of adaptation akin to the stages of adaptation that sojourners experience when entering and adapting to a new unknown culture. If you are a caregiver, it is an experience that will change the way you view the lives around you as well as change your own life.

What's Next? The Shifting Modes of Caregiving

Every cancer situation is different, and caregiving for a family member will probably shift over time, sometimes becoming more intense and demanding, sometimes falling into a predictable routine that feels quite manageable. Some individuals undergoing chemotherapy, for instance, will face hair loss that unnerves them emotionally; the caregiver must account for those emotional upheavals as well as help shave the patient's head, learn to tie headscarves, or schedule a fitting for a wig. Other chemo patients will face nausea that may be mild or severe, that may be predictable in the chemo schedule or come out of the blue; the caregiver will need to help negotiate medications to alleviate side effects as well as clean the patient. Yet other chemo patients will develop sensitivity to cold that requires the caregiver to retrieve items from the refrigerator even if the patient is physically able to walk to and open the refrigerator. Over several months, a patient and caregiver may fall into a routine that is guided by the chemo cycle. Communication changes as circumstances change, and awareness of the need to adapt helps both patient and caregiver work toward shared meaning in unfamiliar situations.

Individuals in the more advanced stages of cancer often experience physical pain and discomfort as symptoms of their illness. The caregiver needs to help manage such discomfort carefully with medication because patients in pain may not be able to keep track of times and dosages themselves. Strong communication and working toward shared meaning can be difficult in such situations and yet can be all the more important for the patient to live the best life possible.

Many patients with late-stage cancer also experience psychological distress directly related to their declining physical conditions as well as their attitudes toward dying. While the caregiver may be able to provide emotional support, the caregiver may also want to contact a healthcare facility or an area church for additional emotional or spiritual guidance for the patient. Each of these shifting situations in the patient affects the caregiver as well, placing new demands mentally, physically, and emotionally and requiring the caregiver to adapt.

In addition, family caregivers are frequently asked to talk about topics they have not thought much about before a cancer diagnosis. The cancer experience opens up a whole new cultural world of different language, terminology, and situations. A daughter may not know how to converse with her father about chemotherapy, radiation, needles, bowel movements, loneliness, personal safety, and intimate care. Such uncomfortable, stressful, socially taboo, and sensitive topics can cause family caregivers and patients to experience periods of awkwardness and embarrassment never before experienced. Different patients will respond to different ways of communicating through such awkwardness.

Humor—between caregiver and patient or between caregiver and others—is one mechanism available to help caregivers manage awkward situations. Humor can be a kind of intimacy and make an uncomfortable situation feel less serious. Caregivers and others, however, should also be leery of offending the patient with humor. The use of humor is incredibly dependent on the specific interaction and individuals.

Caregivers rightly need to maintain the patient's privacy. Caregivers, though, may feel better when they share anecdotes with others to relieve the stress. When Carla Malden (2011) was taking care of her husband at home after he was diagnosed with advanced colorectal cancer, she shared her experiences with her sister in nightly phone calls. This regular conversation with someone other than the patient and healthcare providers was a respite. While neither ignored that Laurence was sick, Malden was grateful that her sister listened as if it were just like any other conversation and as if her husband had some minor ailment.

Caregiver support groups—in person or online—can be especially helpful because the caregiver may find people there who understand the awkward situations and the type of stress, and group members may have suggestions to make situations less awkward and stressful.

Caregiving as Teamwork

Not every patient has a spouse, child, or other family member who can step into the role of caregiver. Healthcare facilities can sometimes help arrange transportation between home and appointments when the patient doesn't have the means. Sometimes caregiving is shared among numerous friends and neighbors, who check in on the patient.

The patient and primary caregiver should talk openly about the roles of others. One helpful way to understand the layers of relationships supporting a patient is discussed by Susan Silk and Barry Goldman (2013) in "How Not To Say the Wrong Thing." This article can help close and distant friends and family consider their roles, so it's the sort of piece a patient or caregiver might post to social media so that friends can read about what the article's authors call the Ring Theory:

> Draw a circle. This is the center ring. In it, put the name of the person at the center of the current trauma. [...] Now draw a larger circle around the first one. In that ring put the name of the person next closest to the trauma. [Often that's the patient's spouse or life partner.] Repeat the process as many times as you need to. In each larger ring put the next closest people. Parents and children before more distant relatives. Intimate friends in smaller rings, less intimate friends in larger ones.

This diagram of rings offers the patient and caregiver a way to negotiate priorities and relationships, especially when energy may be low. Importantly, as a type of communication map, this diagram also suggests how individuals can offer support by directing help and comfort in toward smaller rings and how individuals can complain to or seek support from those in larger rings.

Unlike Lisa, whose story opened this chapter, Ariel Gore had always had a difficult relationship with her quirky mother, which made caregiving tricky when her mother was diagnosed with lung cancer. Ariel was not sure she wanted to take care of her mother, Eve. In addition, Gore (2014), who recounts her story in *The End of Eve*, agreed to help her mother if the family moved to a bigger house in Santa Fe, New Mexico. That meant that, as the caregiving began in earnest, the family did not have many social connections at first. On top of that, sometimes Eve did not want or readily accept her daughter's caregiving efforts.

At one point, Gore sent an email to her mother's friends all over the country asking for help with the caregiving. She was surprised and relieved by the response. "Like a miracle they wrote back. A few of them wrote back, anyway. Yes, maybe they could come. They would check their calendars. Yes, three days or a week? They could probably commit to that. They'd had their hard times with Eve, they said, but they loved her" (p. 184). A mish-mash of her mother's old friends showed up. Gore set up scheduling and notes on a calendar and dry erase board, stocked up on chocolate and wine, and set up videos and music. Gore got the caregiving help she needed, her mother enjoyed rekindling relationships, and the visitors felt as if they were doing a good deed for a friend.

Playwright Eve Ensler (2013) had a different dilemma when she was diagnosed with uterine cancer. She was alone. As more women forego marriage and childbearing, as divorce rates hover around fifty percent, and as husbands are likely to die first among aging opposite-sex couples, this experience may become more common. In her memoir *In the Body of the World*, Ensler (2013) wrote that, at the time of her diagnosis, she did not have that one person on which she could depend to see her through the illness. Her former husband of fifteen years sent an email, a former romantic partner of thirteen years sent a card, and another long-term lover said nothing.

Ensler (2013) was surprised, however, by the extensive support of friends. Her experience demonstrates the range of tasks a caregiver can perform and also the benefits of collaborative caregiving in which the whole becomes more than the sum of its parts, with even small caregiving contributions adding up. One friend cooked eggs that settled her stomach, and another rubbed her feet. Her son returned. Her friend Nico flew back from Italy to stay for a month; he shaved her head. One friend sent silky pajamas, and another spoon fed her soup in the hospital. Numerous friends brought food, gifts, and good company, whether she was feeling good or rotten. "This daily subtle, simple gathering of kindnesses," Ensler (2013) writes, "stretched out across the chemo days and months was, in fact, love" (p. 165). Ensler's experience is unusual because she led a dynamic life of activism that spoke up for others, and then many others returned the favor when she needed care.

While every patient and that patient's social context is different, Ensler's experience speaks to the generosity and collaboration of caregiving that can emerge around a cancer diagnosis.

Caring for Caregivers

As one person in a family provides the care for the cancer patient, other members of the family and friends can step up to take care of the family responsibilities that the patient and the caregiver have been doing, such as laundry, grocery shopping, errands, cleaning, and so on. Caregiving is an issue affecting the entire family. Handling all these shifts in responsibility is rarely easy.

Communication among family members is likely to change when a family member takes on caregiver roles in or outside the home. In this heightened crisis communication situation, communication sometimes improves as a family works together on what has become a shared priority: caregiving for the family member with cancer. But over time, the stress can cause communication breakdowns among family members and introduce stress into what would otherwise be normal conversations. Marital satisfaction can be damaged by the financial, physical, and emotional burdens associated with the new and ongoing caregiving relationship. Among married couples who care for a parent in the same home, some report that the parent's presence constrains time spent on communication within the marital relationship, reduces the amount of private time between couples, and increases time spent on specific types of communication between the couple, including making decisions. Couples who report these shifts also voice lower marital satisfaction (Sparks (Bethea), 2002). Communication within the home and seeking support beyond it can help caregivers manage and help families flourish, but it is not uncomplicated.

In her memoir *The Long Goodbye*, poet Meghan O'Rourke (2011) talks of the toll that her attention to her mother, who had metastatic colon cancer, took on her own romantic relationships. Her mother sometimes felt down and depressed or frightened. Though she had not seen it as a choice, the man she was dating perceived O'Rourke as choosing her mother over him because of O'Rourke's split attention and her mother's needs. Was the man O'Rourke was dating insensitive to her needs, or was she insensitive to his? By the time they talked about how each of them saw the situation and their priorities differently, they had established frustrations and patterns that were difficult to alter.

Various changes in communication during the continuum of cancer care appear to affect even long-term marriages. In her memoir about living with ovarian cancer, literary critic Susan Gubar (2012) writes about her husband's caretaking and how she fretted over what it meant to his life and their relationship:

> I considered the debulked life he now lived—lending me a hand in the shower, bringing me tea, gathering logs for the fireplace, answering the phone with reports of my progress, setting and clearing the table, doing the laundry, tossing dead flowers and gift baskets. I fretted that he had 'been there, done that' decades before and with the steadfast patience he had shown his dying first wife. (p. 90)

Gubar loved her husband, in part, because he was such a caring person, but she worried that the caregiving her cancer demanded took an unreasonable toll on his life. Being aware of and addressing these communication shifts and stresses can be helpful, if somewhat difficult, during caregiving. Even in relationships with strong communication, shared meaning must often be reestablished as circumstances change.

Caregivers often see the patient as never before, and that in itself can be emotionally demanding. Amber, Robin Roberts's (2014) partner and caregiver, recounts in *Everybody's Got Something* watching Roberts try to send email even though she was unable to keep her device in her hand. She witnessed the person she loved writhing in pain, throwing up, and hallucinating from medication. All the while, she told herself that it was a phase. It was a phase, and Amber persevered. Her memories, though, are important touchstones for other caregivers who may be in similar circumstances without knowing others who've been through the caregiving process.

Hospice as Caregiving

Often, when the patient has advanced-stage cancer or when treatment options are limited, a healthcare provider will suggest palliative care or hospice care. A patient or caregiver may want to ask about these options even if the physician does not bring it up in conversation. Some people are uncomfortable with the words *palliative care* and *hospice* as well as with *death*, *dying*, and *end-of-life decisions*. Even though the one certainty of life is that each of us will die, we often have a difficult time talking about these unknown issues and, as a result, tend to ignore their existence as a part of our lives and in our communication with others.

Traditionally, especially in Western medicine, the goal of medical care has been to extend life while, it is always hoped, doing the patient no harm. When cancer is advanced, that becomes a difficult balance to maintain. Palliative care is one of the growing areas of health care designed to address that dilemma. The goal of *palliative care* or *palliative medicine*—sometimes referred to as *comfort care*, *supportive care*, or *symptom management*—is providing quality of life while preventing or treating the symptoms of disease as early as possible. The word *palliative* comes from the Latin word meaning *to cloak*, so that palliative care cloaks, hides, or alleviates various symptoms of the disease. While the cancer may or may not be treatable, the symptoms it causes, including pain, can be managed. Palliative care also involves handling any side effects, including the psychological, social, and spiritual issues that may arise in new ways as the disease progresses.

While in the hospital recovering from unsuccessful surgery to remove the tumor on her pancreas, Mary Lee Leahy (author Anna Leahy's mother) was visited by a palliative care physician, who asked her a range of questions about her life and her current health situation. She was able to talk about what was most important to her in living the best life possible, to prioritize her symptoms, and to convey that she did not want any extraordinary means to extend her life when there was little chance of surviving a year. The physician also talked privately with her daughter to glean more insight in how best to help Mary Lee live the best life possible.

Hospice is defined as a group of professionals and volunteers providing medical, psychological, social, and spiritual care and support to terminally ill individuals and their loved ones. Hospice focuses on quality of life and issues of peace, comfort, and dignity surrounding the death and dying experience as well as bereavement support for the family. Because hospice offers care designed for end-of-life, a hospice home service or facility is likely to require that the patient sign a DNR, or Do-Not-Resuscitate order. In addition, the patient's physician usually must indicate that the patient is unlikely to live more than six months. Some patients, however, live for years in hospice care. In fact, presumably because hospice alleviates both physical pain and mental and emotional stress, hospice patients, according to a study in the *New England Journal of Medicine* (Conner et al., 2007), live several weeks longer than their counterparts who do not partake in hospice care.

When a hospital social worker came into Andy Leahy's (author Anna Leahy's father) hospital room and said that he should consider hospice, he was not prepared for the conversation and became extremely upset. Later that day, his physicians, nurses, and wife talked with him about a hospice facility as an option, and he agreed to consider it because all parties involved had worked toward shared meaning. But within a few days, hospice denied his admittance because, even though he was no longer being actively treated for cancer, a few indicators in his most recent blood test had shown improvement. That was 1986, and hospice and health communication has changed a lot since then. A patient in the same situation today would be able receive hospice care. Communication is necessary to make sure patients and caregivers have a current and accurate understanding of hospice care.

Decades later, when Andy's wife, Mary Lee, was diagnosed with pancreatic cancer, she knew that the time for hospice would come, probably within a year. She had pursued chemotherapy to manage the pain that her tumor caused, and that treatment had undoubtedly extended her life a few months as well. When her oncologist saw that her disease was progressing, he talked with her about home hospice, she expressed her questions about what hospice meant, and her daughter researched area hospice services. A case-managing nurse visited within twenty-four hours of the oncologist's written order and coordinated Mary Lee's care throughout her remaining days. A hospital bed arrived the next day; Mary Lee was more comfortable and, because it could be raised, caregivers' backs got a break. Hospice coordinated all medications with the oncologist, brought supplies to the home, taught the caregivers how to keep Mary Lee comfortable, and provided a crisis kit for caregivers to use when death became imminent. Mary Lee's daughters and sister could call hospice with any questions about care, whether it be physical, emotional, or spiritual. Communication about medical needs and patient comfort was well coordinated.

Many patients with serious, incurable diseases, including late-stage cancer, prefer to die at home like Mary Lee, and the vast majority of people do die at home. Bereaved family members find that the at-home death, along with advanced care planning, is often associated with greater satisfaction (Sparks, 2013). Often, though, this event is a new experience for families, and they will need to seek information. Families and patients needing hospice services at home should turn to the treating physician, to friends whose families have used hospice, and to information about hospice organizations widely available online. Patients, caregivers, and healthcare providers must find ways to talk openly about hospice for it to have the greatest benefit for all individuals involved in a person's cancer care.

Exercise & Discussion

Consider and discuss how the following aspects of cultural and social identity might affect communication between a patient and a potential caregiver(s). You may need to refer to previous chapters to review aspects of cultural and social identity discussed there.

- Age
- Gender
- Ethnicity
- Religion
- Economic class
- Education
- Employment
- Leisure activity
- Personal space preferences
- Attitudes toward time

Now, use the list above to describe your own identity. Then, with this self-awareness, consider how you would make decisions about how to spend your time if you had been diagnosed with cancer and would be undergoing treatment with potentially serious side effects for the next several months. How would you make decisions about how to spend your time if your cancer had a poor prognosis and expected to live one year? How would you communicate your priorities to caregivers, family, and friends?

References

Bevan, J., & Sparks, L. (2011). Communication in the context of long-distance family caregiving: An integrated review and practical applications. *Patient Education and Counseling*, 85, 26–30.

Bevan, J., Vreeburg, S. K., Verdugo, S., & Sparks, L. (2012). Interpersonal conflict and health perception in long-distance caregiving relationships. *Journal of Health Communication*, 1–15. doi:10.1080/10810730.2011.650829

Browne, J. L., & Chan, A. C. (2012). Mother–daughter communication about mammography in an Australian sample. *Journal of Family Communication, 12*(2), 129–150. doi:10.1080/15267431.2011.561144

Connor, S. R., Pyenson B., Fitch K., Spence C., & Iawasaki, K. (2007). Comparing hospice and nonhospice survival among patients who die within a three-year window. *Journal of Pain and Symptom Management, 33*, 238–246.

Ensler, E. (2013). *In the body of the world*. New York, NY: Metropolitan.

Family Caregiver Alliance. (2003). Women and caregiving: Facts and figures. Retrieved from https://www.caregiver.org/women-and-caregiving-facts-and-figures

Fisher, C. L., & Nussbaum, J. F. (2015). Maximizing wellness in successful aging and cancer coping: The importance of family communication from a socioemotional selectivity theoretical perspective. *Journal of Family Communication, 15*, 3–19. doi:10.1080/15267431.2014.946512

Gore, A. (2014). *The end of Eve*. Portland, OR: Hawthorne.

Grigoryeva, A. (2014). When gender trumps everything: The division of parent care among siblings. Center for the Study of Social Organization. Retrieved from https://www.princeton.edu/csso/working-papers/WP9-Grigoryeva.pdf

Gubar, S. (2012). *Memoir of a debulked woman*. New York, NY: W.W. Norton.

Jain, S. L. (2013). *Malignant: How cancer becomes us*. Oakland, CA: University of California Press.

Kamen, C., Mustian, K., Johnson, M., & Boehmer, U. Same-sex couples matter in cancer care. *Journal of Oncology Practice, 11(2)*, 212–215. doi: 10.1200/JOP.2014.000877

Malden, C. (2011). *Afterimage: A brokenhearted memoir of a charmed life*. Guilford, CT: Skirt.

O'Rourke, M. (2011). *The long goodbye*. New York, NY: Riverhead.

Roberts, R. (2014). *Everybody's got something*. New York, NY: Grand Central.

Romm, R. (2009). *The mercy papers: A memoir of three weeks*. New York, NY: Scribner.

Silk, S., & Goldman, B. (2013, April 7). How not to say the wrong thing. *Los Angeles Times*. Retrieved from http://articles.latimes.com/2013/apr/07/opinion/la-oe-0407-silk-ring-theory-20130407

Sparks (Bethea), L. (2002). The impact of an older adult parent on communicative satisfaction and dyadic adjustment in the long-term marital relationship: Adult children and spouses' retrospective accounts. *Journal of Applied Communication Research, 30*, 107–125.

Sparks, L. (2003). An introduction to cancer communication and aging: Theoretical and research insights. *Health Communication, 15*, 123–132.

Sparks, L. (2013). Health communication and caregiving research, policy, and practice. *Caregiving across the professions: A multi-disciplinary, coordinated perspective*. New York, NY: Springer.

· 9 ·

WARRIOR OR CITIZEN?

Metaphors and Messages in Cancer Care

I rose from the gossip and took flight,
and my breath carried me to heights hidden
behind the clouds of that dark day, above birds
crowding in great black flocks in the park.
I knew I had entered forever the world of the ill.
I would never return to that other, open life
of carefree women peeling tangerines.
Sheared off, I was, like the umbilical cord
of my friend's newborn, slashed by her hip bone
as he was pushed too early into a cold birth.

—from "Something Understood" by Anya Silver

When columnist Christopher Hitchens was diagnosed with esophageal cancer, some of the ways his colleagues, friends, and readers talked about his illness irritated him. Even though he surely had heard people talk about other people with cancer in similar ways and though he often understood the thought and emotion behind their words, he heard these phrases as a patient for the first time. They didn't resonate with him. He began thinking about what these messages really meant for the person with cancer.

In his book *Mortality*, Christopher Hitchens (2012) writes, "People don't have cancer: They are reported to be battling cancer. No well-wisher omits the combative image: You can beat this" (p. 6). Hitchens points out some of the metaphors we use to talk about cancer: cancer as war (battling) and cancer as a place. He recognized the prevalence and importance of using metaphors as part of how we view and communicate about cancer. These metaphors and other common types of messages about cancer may be familiar to readers, but they are often under-examined by both scholars and colloquial users.

Metaphors allow individuals to communicate by using a term or phrase to refer to an object or action to which it is not literarily applicable. In addition, metaphors serve as figures of speech that allow participants in an interaction to communicate about abstractions or concepts that are difficult to grasp by employing more concrete or better understood concepts. In this way, using metaphors allows an individual or a group to use commonly understood aspects of a battle or a place to converse about the continuum of cancer care.

This chapter begins with a discussion of messages as they are used to address cancer prevention and treatment. Building on that foundation, the chapter goes on to analyze how framing messages functions over the continuum of cancer care. In the scholarly context of cancer communication, metaphor is then discussed.

Risk Messages

Risk Messages and Healthy Behaviors

Think about some of the conversations you heard when you were a child sitting around the family dinner table. You might recall Mom saying, *eat your vegetables*. You may not have been allowed to drink soda or may have had sweets limited. You may remember fast food as a treat or a stop for a meal when traveling. Some families are more attuned to promoting healthy behaviors of diet and exercise within the family culture than are other families.

For those of us who have experienced cancer within our families, we may be more vigilant in translating healthy messages and behaviors to our children, friends, and others around us in subtle and sometimes not so subtle ways. Lisa Sparks's father died of lung cancer—with 16 additional brain metastases—in 1997 at the age of just 58. Although he had not smoked in the last ten years of his life, he had started smoking at the age of 15 and continued smoking off and on throughout most of his adult life. Lisa (one of this book's authors) has never been a smoker and has always been sensitive to smoke in the air because of allergies. So, throughout her entire life, she has avoided even secondhand smoke. Now, she passes down persuasive health messages and behaviors about the risks of smoking to her family members. In fact, health risk messages related to diet, exercise, and sunscreen protection are sometimes topics for discussion at her family dinner table. Her experiences with people who have had cancer and her understanding of risk affect her day-to-day interactions with others.

Every family creates a family culture, and Lisa fosters a culture of healthy behaviors in which risk messages and behaviors become integrated into family life. Of course, not every day is filled with perfect health behavior, but the goal is for the family to consistently engage in more healthy behaviors and choices than not and for those healthy behaviors to become habits that everyone takes for granted. It is not always easy to make healthy choices, but when healthy behaviors become an embedded part of everyday life, they are more likely to stick across a person's lifespan, including during cancer care.

These cues and reminders about healthy behaviors and consequences are called *risk messages*. The ways individuals process risk messages are a part of our human physiology. In other words, we are hard-wired to think about risk in certain ways, and we process risk—sometimes without consciously thinking much about it—to make decisions. What happens when you think you see a snake on the ground? Your immediate reaction may be to scream and point or to move back quickly. Or you may freeze in fear. Your brain sees an image, and your body responds almost automatically. Our physical response to the snake is driven by how we view perceived risks.

Perceived risk is physiological, so it is possible to understand some expected patterns of behavior in response to risk. Certain types of risk messages—like *eat your vegetables*—create certain types of responses, so it is really important to convey risk in ways that encourage healthy behaviors. Sometimes a lecture on the benefits of green leafy vegetables, for instance, is not the best way to convince children to gobble up healthy food instead of snacks and fast food carefully designed to entice them.

Risk Messages and Cancer Prevention

Communication about risk is important in the context of cancer for two crucial reasons.

1) Communication about risk is vital to prevention of cancer. How can we best communicate information about the risks of smoking, sun exposure, poor diet, lack of exercise, or unprotected sex to encourage habits that will lower a person's risk of cancer?

At least one-half of all deaths in the United States can be attributed to preventable behavioral and social factors, such as poor diets, smoking, alcohol use, and poor environmental health conditions. These numbers are in line with similar statistics from other first-world nations (World Health Organization [WHO], 2016). Behaviors associated with increased risk for cancers have been consistently linked to mortality rates, but oftentimes people do not consider the potentially hazardous outcomes of such behaviors.

In other words, though Christopher Hitchens's father died of esophageal cancer, Christopher himself engaged in behaviors like smoking and drinking that increased his own risk of the same cancer. He likely socialized with others who engaged in the same unhealthy behaviors too. Often, it seems easier to continue behavior than to change behavior, to continue to fit in rather than upset the status quo or fail at the change. The more immediate fear of losing one's social status often seems greater, and fear of social upheaval or fear of failure often wins out over behavior we know is better for us. Understanding how we perceive immediate and long-term reward and risk can help us communicate effectively so that individuals feel more capable of making good decisions for their health.

Risk Messages and Cancer Treatment

The second reason that communication of risk is important applies more immediately to the readers of this book and to making decisions about cancer care.

2) Communication of risk is important in cancer treatment or therapy. Each treatment option—whether it be surgery, chemotherapy, radiation, or something else—carries its own risks, some of which may be mild and some of which may be life threatening. In addition, those

> risks may vary from situation to situation. How can we communicate information about risk to people who must decide whether a particular treatment option is worth it for their situation?

Even though each cancer treatment carries significant risk, it is easy to see why a person will put up with many of those risks when facing a serious health crisis. Chemotherapy can nausea, neuropathy, hair loss, numerous needle sticks, long infusion appointments, additional invasive tests, heart damage, and even life-threatening allergic reactions. But our fear of cancer—and of metastasis (or spread of cancer) or of death from cancer—often, though certainly not always, outweighs the fear associated with a given treatment.

Some people do not feel this way about a particular treatment option. Instead, they fear the treatment more than the cancer. Many factors influence therapy decisions, including age, general health, family relationships, financial circumstances, and so on. As a result, a young woman who plans to start a family may fear infertility caused by a certain treatment, or someone without health insurance may fear exorbitant costs of treatment.

In addition, the potential benefits may vary. The bigger the potential payoff, the more comfortable many people are gambling with risks or side effects. The same chemotherapy may be curative for one patient and palliative for another, and the patient who perceives a potential cancer-free life may be willing to assume more risk in treatment than the terminally ill patient. Some people choose not to undergo certain therapies because the treatment seems more debilitating than the cancer or will not make a significant enough difference to them in the quantity or quality of their lives.

Understanding risk messages and how they apply to the patient's situation can help a person make better decisions. When it comes to cancer care, there often exists no completely good or completely bad choice. There exists no simple formula for risk assessment that works across all patients. Instead, patients must sort through the pros and cons, understand and try to balance immediate and long-term fears, and weigh the risks for themselves to make decisions.

Prospect Theory: Framing the Message to Make Decisions

Hidden Meaning: How Information Is Framed

Health communication scholars have been trying to understand how cancer patients make decisions. In recent years, some have come to the realization that presenting information within a frame—or a context—of gains and losses is crucial to how individuals make decisions, especially with decisions that have significant risk. We call this way of understanding communication and decision-making *prospect theory*. The word *prospect* comes from Latin words that mean *to look ahead* or *to see through*. It is difficult to look ahead when you are in the midst of cancer care, but paying attention to framing can help you sort through information for hidden meaning that many patients are not usually able to see when they communicate with healthcare providers, scour the Internet for information, or seek informal advice.

People encode information or put information into a context when they share it—that is typically referred to as *framing the message*. In addition, people make choices in terms of potential gains or potential losses they perceive in that message. In other words, frames are meaning added to information, and frames can be altered without changing the factual information. The same factually equivalent information can be presented in different ways. The message can be framed or encoded by either a gain or a loss, by either a positive or a negative context.

Some health communication scholars and health practitioners who attempt to understand the communication involved in risky decisions have used message framing to apply prospect theory to the questions involved (see e.g., Kahneman & Tversky, 1979, 2000; Sparks, 2007, 2011, 2013; Sparks & Villagran, 2010; Tversky & Kahneman, 1981). The landmark essays of Amos Tversky and Daniel Kahneman (1979, 2000) describe prospect theory, which suggests that individuals will respond differentially depending on whether information is presented in relation to gains or losses. People hearing or reading information that is relevant to the decision they face encode that information in terms of potential gains or potential losses embedded in the message's frame. "We use the term 'decision frame' to refer to the decision-maker's conception of the acts, outcomes, and contingencies associated with a particular choice. The frame that a decision-maker adopts is controlled partly by the formulation of the problem and partly by the norms, habits, and personal characteristics of the decision-maker" (Tversky & Kahneman, 1981, p. 453). Further, Entman (1991) asserted that framing is the process of selecting a particular aspect of an issue to make it more salient in a shared message. This process of framing, which is discussed in *Health Communication in the 21st Century* (Wright, Sparks, & O'Hair, 2013), promotes a particular definition among potential definitions, a particular viewpoint or perspective among ways of seeing the issue, a particular interpretation among several ways to understand the issue, a particular moral evaluation, and/or a particular treatment recommendation among the options available.

The standard, textbook example of a framing problem in health communication is the lives-saved-lives-lost question. Let's look at a choice between two hypothetical public health programs proposed to deal with an epidemic that is threatening 600 lives. One program emphasizes that the program will certainly save 200 lives. The other program has a 1/3 chance of saving all 600 lives and a 2/3 chance of saving none. In this version, more people prefer the program that will save 200 lives for sure. Two-hundred lives sound like a lot, and people like to bet on sure things.

But let's look at the same information put a different way. In the second version of the factual information, the first program could result in 400 deaths. This is rather simple math; if 200 of 600 lives are certainly saved, that means 400 might be lost. The second option, put another way, has a 2/3 chance of 600 deaths and a 1/3 chance of no deaths. Again, the facts remain the same, but the information focuses on negative consequences. When the information is framed this way, most people prefer the gamble and opt for the second program (e.g., Sparks, 2013).

These two formulations present identical information. Only the frame has changed. In the first formulation, the problem is framed in terms of lives *saved*; in the second, the problem is framed as a matter of lives *lost*. One version focuses on gains, and the other, on losses. That change in focus alters people's interpretations of the facts. Individuals tend to select and emphasize some aspects of a perceived reality and make them more salient during an interaction or exchange of information. Thus, the message frame—the way of understanding the problem—that a decision-maker uses is controlled, in part, by how the problem has been framed. In addition, the norms, habits, and personal characteristics of the decision-maker further interpret the encoded information.

Nearly all health-related information can be construed in terms either of gains or of losses, of benefits or of costs. But which frame works better? The answer depends on whether the target health behavior is an illness-protection behavior or an illness-detection behavior.

Protection behaviors, like using sunscreen or seatbelts, typically lead to somewhat more certain outcomes, and the act does not give you new information about your health. In these instances, you are more likely to maintain your current healthy status if you perform these behaviors. Gain-framed information leads to preference for certainty. Therefore, gain-framed messages that emphasize benefits—lives saved or increase in life expectancy—are effective in promoting infant car restraints, physical exercise, smoking cessation, and sunscreen (Sparks, 2013). *Gain-framed information* works more like the carrot than the stick, pointing out the likely reward for a protection behavior.

Prostate exams, mammography, mole exams—these are detection behaviors. In these examples, the individual is seeking information and may—or may not—find something wrong. Prospect theory predicts that loss-framed information leads to preference for or comfort with uncertainty—maybe or maybe not—and encourages patients to get a screening test. In other words, health information like informing a woman that 1 in 7 women are diagnosed with breast cancer in their lives tends to use potential loss to encourage detection behaviors, in this case a mammogram. *Loss-framed information* works a little like scare tactics—the stick instead of the carrot—that make clear the threat to your health if you do not engage in the behavior.

Every health communication scholar cares about how messages are framed positively and negatively, and the provider, patient, and caregiver should care as well. Information is power. Framing recasts information, funneling its power toward one direction or another. When a patient more deeply understands how information about one's cancer and treatment options are being framed, that patient can make better decisions for the situation. When a patient asks the oncologist about the chance that chemotherapy will be successful, does the answer emphasize how many people's tumors shrink—the great benefit—or its failure rate? When the patient asks the oncologist about the likelihood of a particular side effect of chemotherapy, perhaps nausea or neuropathy, does that patient get information about how many people experience that side effect or how many do not experience it or do not think it is severe? Does the physician talk about how rare this type of cancer is for the patient's age or how many patients that age the physician has treated for this type of cancer?

Consider whether the way information that is presented emphasizes gains, benefits, or positive outcomes or emphasizes losses, risks, or negative outcomes.

Rephrasing information in a different frame can help a person see whether the frame gives the facts different weight. In other words, pay attention not only to the factual information but also to how that information is presented.

How Framing Shapes Caregiving

A family member or caregiver may be able to use some persuasive techniques described here—especially framing in terms of benefits or losses—while caring for cancer patients, whether in a stage of cancer prevention, detection, diagnosis, treatment, survivorship, or possibly at end-of-life.

Many people view asking for help—whether a ride to a doctor appointment or accepting hospice care—as a sign of weakness. Help or caregiving, though, can be reframed because it is also a way for the patient to remain strong. While sometimes exhausted by the task, caregivers gain strength, too, through the important, rewarding work they do as caregivers. Rarely does only one way of looking at—framing—information or a situation reveal all the potential benefits and costs. And sometimes, though losses may be great, a few small gains make all the difference in a person's life.

Let's consider an example from end-of-life decision-making. The patient—let's say she is your mother—has exhausted all reasonable treatment options. Her options are more limited than they have been over the past year. Perhaps, she cannot tolerate any more chemotherapy because of side effects, or maybe treatment is no longer effective in controlling the growth and spread of the cancer, so more treatment wouldn't be worth the side effects even if your mother could tolerate more of the drugs. (That was the situation for Anna Leahy's mother and a reason she became interested in writing this book.) Let's say she is not eligible for clinical trials either because the criteria are often very narrow; maybe your mother's diabetes makes her ineligible, or she has received a treatment drug that would confuse the results of a study of a different drug. You have been doing a good job of taking care of your mother, but you are barely able to meet her healthcare needs right now, and you know she is growing weaker. You worry that you are not up for the task alone, and the doctor suggests hospice as an option for supportive care. But your mother thinks of hospice as only for the very end of life, perhaps when a patient is bed-ridden or barely conscious. Maybe she wants to continue fighting the battle and worries that hospice will require her to take more pain medication that clouds her thinking or to give up altogether. Or maybe, even though she has come to terms with the prognosis, she doesn't want to see herself as more helpless or dependent.

She is not wrong in her concerns, and you may share some of her concerns and think you are selfish for wanting to lessen your own caregiving burden by sharing it with others. But she has used only a negative frame to understand hospice care. Instead, the patient and the caregiver can frame the problem positively, emphasizing the benefits—that someone will visit to wash her hair, that hospice will allow her to stay in her own home, that some patients live longer and are more alert in hospice, that hospice caregivers have expertise that informal caregivers may not have. This new frame accentuates other ways to think about hospice, including possible gains for the patient as well as for the caregiver. Hospice remains the patient's decision, but the information she has and the frame through which she interprets the information influence her decision.

Metaphors: How We Talk About Our Relationship to Cancer

While communication between physicians and patients often depends most heavily on medical terminology and modes of conversation that focus on the biomedical approach to cancer care, we also have colloquial, conversational, or cultural ways of talking about cancer. Metaphors are often woven through conversations that those with cancer have with family, friends, and even healthcare professionals. We usually do not think explicitly about the metaphors and messages we use, but they often reveal our attitudes. Patients and caregivers should consider consciously the ways they choose to refer to cancer, cancer treatment, and cancer patients. In doing this, they can more actively set the terms and tone for their interactions with others.

Cancer as Place: Territory and Citizenship in Cancer Land

Susan Sontag (1977), in her book *Illness as a Metaphor,* talked of illness as a place we sometimes live. "Illness is the night-side of life, a more onerous citizenship. Everyone who is born holds dual citizenship, in the kingdom of the well and in the kingdom of the sick. Although we all prefer to use only the good passport, sooner or later each of us is obliged, at least for a spell, to identify ourselves as citizens of that other place" (p. 3). Consider what it means when we think of cancer this way. Perhaps, for instance, thinking of cancer as a place makes patients feel greater control over how they negotiate the landscape of cancer organizations. Learning about cancer and treatment can feel like learning to find one's way around a foreign land or adapt to a new environment. Information and communication can work like a map for making one's way through the cancer experience.

Christopher Hitchens (2012) also described his early days with cancer using the same kind of metaphor of place and citizenship. At first, he tried to be, at least metaphorically, two places at once: "I managed to pull off both gigs without anyone noticing anything amiss, though I did vomit two times, with an extraordinary combination of accuracy, neatness, violence, and profusion, just before each show. This is what citizens of the sick country do while they are still hopelessly clinging to their old domicile" (pp. 2–3). He also described some of the ways he assimilated: "This new land is quite welcoming in its way. [...] The country has a language of its own—a lingua franca that manages to be both dull and difficult and that contains names like ondansetron, for nausea medication—as well as some unsettling gestures that require a bit of getting used to" (p. 3). These passages echo some of the ideas discussed in Chapter 3 and Chapter 4, where culture and social identity were explored in relation to health communication.

If we are citizens in Cancer Land, we belong there and play a role in what happens. Belonging gives us a sense of how we fit into the larger society. Physicians, then, are akin to the cancer country's officials, people who enforce the land's policies. And the medical language—*tissue*, *palpable*, *mestastasized*—is what Hitchens (2012) calls "the local Tumorville tongue" (p. 4). Citizens are expected to learn both what to say and how to say it in order to develop useful relationships in this new geography.

Some patients may live in this new territory the rest of their lives, while others will return to the kingdom of the well. If the prognosis is poor, a patient may find the metaphor of cancer as a place comforting. If the prognosis is good, a patient may find this metaphor useful because it suggests a visit, like a tourist. Some patients, however, may not find this way of talking about cancer or illness as a place helpful.

Cancer as Journey

Cancer as a journey is related to the idea of cancer as a place but shifts emphasis from cancer as a state of being to cancer as a process through which a person moves. A patient who talks about cancer as a journey may be especially eager to gather information, to build endurance or patience, or to take action. The journey also suggests that patients themselves learn, grow, or change from the experience, perhaps becoming internally wiser or stronger or taking in stride unexpected detours in treatment.

A patient may also extend this travel metaphor so that a treatment plan functions like an itinerary for a trip with a planned destination of restored health. Some patients may even want to document their experiences with a sort of travel diary or album in social media, which we discuss in Chapter 10. As with any metaphorical way of talking about cancer, some patients and some healthcare providers may find the journey analogy useful, whereas others may not.

Cancer as War: Variation on the Theme

Cancer as war is probably the most widely accepted metaphor in cancer conversations. Many people, in fact, gain strength by thinking about and talking about cancer as a battle they are waging against an enemy or, especially perhaps for children, against a monster. In fact, the battle metaphor is probably the most well-known and widely accepted way of describing a person's relationship with cancer. Gilda Radner (2009) wrote about her long fight this way: "I saw cancer as a battle, as a hell, as tortures" (p. 203). As one reads her account of "battling cancer," her attitude and language may go unnoticed because this approach seems completely appropriate to her circumstances as a cancer patient.

This battle metaphor comes with an organized plan—a way of thinking and talking—that a patient or a physician can apply to the patient's relationship with cancer in a variety of situations. As Siddhartha Mukherjee (2010) pointed out, using both the personification of cancer as an enemy and the idea of the human body as territory in *The Emperor of All Maladies:*

> Cancer is an expansionist disease; it invades through tissues, sets up colonies in hostile environments, seeking 'sanctuary' in one organ and then immigrating to another. It lives desperately, inventively, fiercely, territorially, cannily, and defensively—at times teaching *us* how to survive. (p. 38)

Here, the biomedical reality of cancer development and progression of the disease is described through a metaphor instead of with medical terminology.

If cancer patients wage battles, no wonder Mukherjee (2010) wrote of his patient Carla, "But she had made it; a charring, private war had just ended.

[…] I handed her the azaleas and she stood looking at them speechlessly, almost numb from the enormity of her victory" (p. 448). The physical and emotional difficulty of the battle with cancer can make the reward of living all the more welcome and meaningful. Patients and providers can feel empowered by using this metaphor.

Christopher Hitchens (2012) also wrote about cancer as war, but that metaphor troubled him. He found that he had a complex relationship with cancer and that he didn't always feel like a warrior and certainly didn't choose to enter his battle as a soldier. In a sort of compromise with this metaphor, he said, "I'm not fighting or battling cancer—it's fighting me" (p. 89).

Like Hitchens, Susan Gubar (2012) also struggled with this metaphor of cancer as a war in her book *Memoir of a Debulked Woman*. She understood its power and usefulness but was concerned about what this view and language meant for her. "Cancer patients dedicated to an epic struggle against their disease reject any 'surrender' to it as an act 'of conspiring' with it" (p. 29). Her concern, then, is that a patient may not be in a position to fight and that acceptance of the serious nature of the disease should not be judged as failure on the part of the patient.

Gubar admires courage and resolve as part of a patient's goal to survive but cannot muster the optimism she sees in many others with ovarian cancer. She goes on to explain a less optimistic viewpoint: "Other people, because of the advanced stage of their disease or their age or their refusal to put on 'the rose-tinted spectacles' of redemptive narratives, may agree with me that no amount of fighting 'can give you back your life,' that it would be a lie 'to live as though cancer will never return,' and that therefore it is necessary to find a way out of the proposition that if you are not hopefully battling cancer, you are somehow rooting for it" (p. 29). Again, she expresses concern about admiring one patient's optimism and resolve if it means that another patient might be blamed for a pragmatic approach to life with cancer or for the progression of the disease.

In other words, Susan Gubar understands that different metaphors help different people talk about their cancer. Thinking about cancer as a war you fight can be empowering, especially when treatment is going well or you have a difficult treatment step to take, but some patients may feel especially overwhelmed—besieged and beleaguered—when they feel as if they are losing that war, even though they are doing everything they can to become well.

Some people, like Gubar, feel as if the battle metaphor does not ring true to their experiences and as if it places an extra burden on patients, asking those who are in tough situations to show only strength and no weakness. Though she could not articulate it at the time, Lucy Grealy (2003) felt pressure to live up to her mother's expectation that she be brave and not cry. In *Autobiography of a Face*, she describes how she was sometimes unable to keep herself from crying when she faced tremendous discomfort, showing weakness that any child might rightly express. Eve Ensler (2013), who wrote *In the Body of the World*, struggled with the battle metaphor because the cancer was inside of her, and her own body's cells had made the tumor, so she worried that to battle cancer was to be at war with herself.

Ensler (2013), however, revised—with the help of her friend Sue—the metaphor to suit her own views and needs as a cancer patient. Sue explained that the chemotherapy, not Ensler, was doing battle:

> Your job is to welcome the chemo as an empathetic warrior, who is coming to rescue your innocence by killing off the perpetrator who got inside you. [...] When you feel nauseous or terrible, just imagine how hard the chemo is fighting on your behalf and on behalf of all women's bodies, restoring wholeness, innocence, peace. (p. 113)

This metaphorical rendering is not completely accurate to the biomedical reality, since more side effects or side effects of greater severity are not correlated with chemotherapy's efficacy. In this revised version of the battle, however, Ensler was not fighting cancer. Instead, she was allowing other warriors—chemotherapy, for instance—to fight the battle on her behalf. It is a slight but important difference in how she thought about the relationship she had with her cancer and with her cancer treatment. "I think yes, chemo will be my medicine," she wrote. "I will ride it like a lion. I will let it do its work in me."

Common metaphors people use to talk about cancer:

- Geographical Place or Territory
- Journey
- War or Battle

Consider the following questions related to ways of talking about cancer that both reflect and fashion the social reality of cancer care:

- ➢ What does it mean for Susan Sontag assert that healthy people live in "the kingdom of the well"?
- ➢ If life is thought of as a journey, what is the role of cancer in the lifespan?

- In 1999, *The Onion* published a satire story that critiques of the battle metaphor for cancer. Read "Loved Ones Recall Local Man's Cowardly Battle with Cancer" online to consider the implications of using the war metaphor. Do you think this story is funny? Why or why not? http://www.theonion.com/article/loved-ones-recall-local-mans-cowardly-battle-with-772
- The National Cancer Act of 1971 was dubbed the beginning of the War on Cancer. More recently, the Recovery Act of 2009 included funding for cancer research; President Barack Obama wrote the following: "Now is the time to commit ourselves to waging a war against cancer as aggressive as the war cancer wages against us" (Lennon, 2003). How is a national war on cancer different and similar to an individual's battle with cancer?
- In 2015, Emily Phillips penned her own obituary before she died, less than a month after she was diagnosed with pancreatic cancer. Read her obituary online, and peruse others. How does the language of an obituary function as social action? http://www.legacy.com/obituaries/timesunion/obituary.aspx?n=emily-debrayda-phillips&pid=174524066&
- What other metaphors might be used to talk about the disease, the treatment, or the patient when we converse with cancer?

Choosing Your Metaphor

Each patient must use or create the metaphors that convey his or her attitudes best and work toward positive outcomes in cancer care. One patient may gain strength from thinking of oneself as a warrior against cancer, whereas another may think of the healthcare providers or even the treatments themselves as those who are waging the war on behalf of the patient. Still another patient may see cancer as a doppelgänger, a monster, or a shadow. And another may think of cancer as one of many of life's possible paths.

Actively considering which ways of talking about cancer fit a patient's attitudes, priorities, and identities will help the overall communication with others about the person's condition. When others pick up the communicative cues—metaphors—the patient reveals, they are likely to be more comfortable in a variety of interactions with the patient over time. Healthcare providers and caregivers may consider becoming more cognizant of when a patient's metaphors do not match their own preferred ways of talking so that they can adjust and work toward shared meaning.

Negotiating Metaphors and Messages

Although metaphors can sometimes backfire or not properly fit the situation at hand, metaphors, like cancer as a battle or a place, and risk messages can play an important role in facilitating effective cancer communication. Most people—patients, caregivers, family and friends, even healthcare providers—do not often give a great deal of thought to metaphors and risk messages even though everyone uses them on a regular basis. Becoming more aware of ways of talking about cancer and making active choices about how to talk about—and how not to talk about—cancer can help everyone involved in care share information and work toward shared meaning and common goals.

Exercise & Discussion

Keeping Prospect Theory in mind, it may be useful for a cancer patient to do an old-fashioned Pro/Con chart for decision making, whether they be major decisions, like whether to have surgery, or something less directly related to one's physical health.

We have started a chart here with some made-up examples. Because the benefits and risks are different for each type and stage of cancer, each treatment, and each patient, we made up sample information for chemotherapy. Patients would need to adapt the exercise to suit real individual situations and needs.

Remember to (1) *list all the information you can think of related to that particular decision* and (2) *mark the gain or loss that seems most important*. For example, for some patients, the possible benefit that chemotherapy lowers the chance of metastasis may be the most important piece of information to use in the decision, even though there may be more risks listed than benefits. In other words, both quality—weight or importance of information—and quantity matter in decision-making.

Consider Prospect Theory as you add more examples to your chart (as we did in the second row). In other words, you will need to frame the *same* piece of information both positively and negatively. Doing this can help you see that there exists no truly right or wrong decision, only the decision that seems best to the patient in the particular situation at the time. Use this chart to think through five patient decisions, and add others if you prefer.

Decision	Positive (Benefits, Gains)	Negative (Costs, Losses)
Chemotherapy	Tumor Shrinkage, Lowers Chance of Metastasis	Hair Loss, Nausea, Neuropathy, Fatigue, Long Infusion Appointments
Chemotherapy (and some Prospect Theory)	Shrinks Tumor in 20% of Patients, 1 of Every 2 Patients Has No Severe Side Effects	Fails to Shrink Tumor in 80% of Patients, Half the Patients Have Severe Side Effects
Getting a Wig		

References

Ensler, E. (2013). *In the body of the world*. New York, NY: Metropolitan.

Entman, R. M. (1991). Framing: Towards clarification of a fractured paradigm. *Journal of Communication*, *43*, 51–58.

Grealy, L. (2003). *Autobiography of a face*. New York, NY: Harper Perennial.

Gubar, S. (2012). *Memoir of a debulked woman*. New York, NY: W.W. Norton.

Hitchens, C. (2012). *Mortality*. New York, NY: Twelve (Hachett).

Kahneman, D., & Tversky, A. (1979). "Prospect theory:" An analysis of decision under risk. *Econometrica*, *47*, 263–291.

Kahneman, D., & Tversky, A. (2000). *Choices, values, and frames*. New York, NY: Cambridge University Press.

Lennon, C. (2003). Ovarian cancer: Fighting for a cure. *Harper's* 3 June 2009. Retrieved from http://www.harpersbazaar.com/beauty/health/news/a391/barack-obama-ovarian-cancer.

Mukherjee, S. (2010). *The emperor of all maladies*. New York, NY: Scribner.

Radner, G. (1989/2009). *It's always something*. New York, NY: Simon & Schuster.

Sontag, S. (1977). *Illness as metaphor and AIDS and its metaphors*. New York, NY: Picador.

Sparks, L. (2007). Cancer care and the aging patient: Complexities of age-related communication barriers. In H. D. O'Hair, G. L. Kreps, & L. Sparks (Eds.), *Handbook of communication and cancer care* (pp. 233–249). Cresskill, NJ: Hampton Press.

Sparks, L. (2011). *Health risk messages and decision-making: Age-related trends in utilization of the internet and electronic communication devices for coordination of cancer care in elderly patients*. TEDx OrangeCoast, Renee and Henry Segerstrom Concert Hall, Costa Mesa, CA. Retrieved from http://www.youtube.com/watch?v=d4JNyyuonko

Sparks, L. (2013). Health communication and caregiving research, policy, and practice. In R. C. Talley & S. S. Travis (Eds), *Caregiving across the professions: A multi-disciplinary, coordinated perspective* (pp. 131–175). New York, NY: Springer.

Sparks, L., & Villagran, M. (2010). *Patient and provider interaction: A global health communication perspective*. Cambridge: Polity Press.

Tversky, A., & Kahneman, D. (1981). The framing of decisions and the psychology of choice. *Science, 211*, 453–458.

World Health Organization. (2007). *Unequal, unfair, ineffective and inefficient gender inequity in health.* Report by the women and gender equity knowledge network. Geneva, Switzerland. Retrieved from http://www.who.int/social_determinants/resources/csdh_media/wgekn_final_report_07.pdf?ua=1

Wright, K. B., Sparks, L., & O'Hair, H. D. (2013). *Health communication in the 21st century* (2nd ed.). Hoboken, NJ: Wiley & Sons.

· 10 ·

CAN YOU HEAR ME NOW?

Technology and Communication in Cancer Care

When a strong sister phones you with a weak voice,
you know before you know.
Why her? She's five years younger than you.

You want to flip back the calendar to yesterday
when it was bad enough a friend had colon cancer,
when you clinked glasses to your brother's
clean, three-year scan.

You're at the age where the C-word terrorizes: A bomb
could hide in anyone's vest. You begin peering
into the bathroom mirror: Does your skin look yellow?
At night in bed your fingers search your breasts.

Your sister endures the bullet's removal,
then radiation five days times six weeks,
a bad sunburn on her breast, exhaustion.
Tests show she needs no more—
no wig, no Tamoxifen—
she has the "best" kind of cancer.

—from "Diagnosis" by Karen Paul Holmes

Today I shaved my head. Not with a razor but with an electric hair trimmer. [...] So I took the comb off and shaved it down. It left maybe 1/20th of a millimeter. It was the only way to salvage a teeny bit of hair and not reveal the patchiness the radiation has caused. (I was hoping for a suave Jason Stratham look. Not to be.) I then used the same length on my beard. If you've ever seen a movie star with a neat and tidy three-day growth of beard, he's probably used a technique something like this.

I wasn't too displeased although you can really see the scar from the surgery. I was proud to hear [my son] Zeke say that the new haircut made the scar more "prominent" citing that as the one thing he didn't like about it. "Prominent." Nice word. But he's such a nice guy he told me it looked good, Dad.

At first [my daughter] Josephine was scared. Then a little frustration set in when she couldn't see her reflection in it. Then she got used to it. This evening when I was lying next to her while she was supposedly reading Esperanza Rising she said to me: "You know your haircut isn't really that bad. It's kind of nice how you left a little beard. Makes it flow from your face to your head. The only thing is the new haircut makes your ears stick out. You know, your hair really did a good job of hiding those ears. You couldn't even really tell they were stick-out ears."

Like many cancer patients, Adam Schmitz used computer-mediated communication during his cancer care. This excerpt is from his private journal—a blog—at Caring Bridge, and he also used email and social media like Facebook to talk with others about his cancer and keep in touch with his friends while he was ill. These exchanges—mediated communication instead of in-person conversation—gave Adam ways to sort through information, document his physical symptoms, and express his emotional state.

The rise in technology has changed the medical aspect of cancer care with such innovations as digital imaging of CT scans and electronic medical records. Computers have also changed the ways in which patients converse with and about cancer. Some forms of *computer-mediated communication* are interactive and some are not. In other words, some provide a back-and-forth exchange, whereas others provide one-way communication to a passive receiver. Technology-mediated communication can be one person searching for a particular piece of information, like an oncologist checking CT scan results, or it can be a group of geographically distant individuals coming together in virtual space. The continuum of cancer care—from prevention, detection, and diagnosis to treatment, survivorship, and end-of-life—is represented, enacted, and discussed every day through computer-mediated communication.

This chapter gives an overview of how cancer patients might engage in computer-mediated communication about their care and suggests ways both patients and providers can use such communication to improve interactions and outcomes.

Telemedicine

Telemedicine refers to the use of technology as a mode of communication between provider and patient that allows individuals who are not geographically close to their healthcare providers to acquire diagnosis and treatment. Telemedicine is a practical way for patients who live in rural areas and those who are too sick to travel to see specialists and to access health care. Health care can be delivered via various forms of technology, including phones and computers.

Some hospitals, for instance, have a tele-nurse. That way, a patient can talk with a healthcare professional to seek advice without making an appointment. Perhaps, the patient is suffering extreme nausea from chemotherapy, and the doctor's office is closed. The caregiver concerned about dehydration can call the tele-nurse, who can go over symptoms and recommend whether the patient should go to the Emergency Room. Some hospitals do not have a real-time tele-nurse but do have a library of pre-recorded messages that provide information about specific health conditions.

Some providers use a system in which they make an audio recording for a specific patient that can be accessed by calling a phone number and entering a code specific to that patient. This system allows the providers to disseminate information such as test results quickly to multiple patients. If the patient has questions or requires follow-up care, the patient is responsible for contacting the provider. While this system may burden some patients, it allows confidential information to be conveyed to the patient even when provider and patient are not available at the same time for a more interactive phone call.

One of the most widely known and unusual examples of telemedicine in practice is the story of the doctor in Antarctica who needed to treat herself for breast cancer when she could not return to a hospital elsewhere. Jerri Nielson, an emergency room physician, traveled to Antarctica to work at the Amundson-Scott South Pole Station. When she discovered a lump in her breast, she used both email and real-time video-conferencing to seek advice and guidance from experts in the United States so that she could perform a biopsy on herself. The equipment at the medical station was not advanced enough to make a clear diagnosis, so medical supplies were dropped from a plane so that she could retest the excised breast tissue, confirm the cancer diagnosis, and begin treatment with hormone therapy and chemotherapy. Until the weather was good enough to evacuate her several months later, Nielson continued to use the satellite link to communicate with her healthcare advisors thousands of miles away. The self-treatment treatment in the Antarctic and subsequent treatment, including surgery, in the United States was successful, though Nielson's cancer recurred seven years later. Nielson continued to give motivational speeches even after the recurrence of cancer.

Electronic Medical Records

Electronic medical records (EMRs), or electronic health records (EHRs), can be stored and accessed via remote locations through the use of computers, so it is a form of computer-mediated communication. When all individuals on the cancer care team keep electronic medical records, all individuals on that team have access to all the records. In other words, if you have a CT scan at the hospital, you can be at your oncologist's office later that same day looking at the images together on a computer screen. Or when you see a cardiologist to check your heart health before surgery, your surgeon can access those results as soon as they are available.

Electronic medical records communicate a patient's vital information to providers who access them, so this system can be an efficient way to coordinate care among providers, no matter how far they are from each other. In addition, this system can eliminate the need for cancer patients, their families, and their caregivers to provide lengthy descriptions of previous diagnoses and treatments every time a new provider joins the cancer care team or needs an update. Each provider can read all the pertinent information on a given patient in a centralized database. While interactions with patients themselves are important too, a common record helps to ensure everyone on the healthcare team has the same, most complete information. This type of record-keeping is quickly becoming standard throughout healthcare systems in the United States.

In addition, as Lisa Sparks and Michelle Miller-Day discuss in their research, the switch to electronic medical records "has enhanced the amount and quality of health data potentially available to health research [...]. The information generated by EHRs [electronic health records] can be extremely valuable to study and address disparities," (Sparks & Miller-Day, 2014) which may result from poor communication, cultural stereotyping, and other non-medical aspects of health care. In other words, studying large sets of records can help health researchers and health communication scholars recognize patterns and address systemic problems across individual patients or providers.

Internet Information

Internet information is an example of computer-mediated communication designed as *mass-mediated communication*, or communication of the same information to everyone who accesses it. The Internet has become an important channel for providers and organizations to communicate with patients and each other, a source for social support among patients, and a means for health campaigns to reach individuals around the world. Because of the Internet, more health information is more accessible to more people than at any other time in history. One study indicated that, among individuals who use the Internet, as many as 8 out of 10 individuals seek health information online. Typically, people searching for health information about cancer look for material about cancer prevention, diagnosis, specific types of cancer, and both traditional and experimental cancer treatment options (Kreps et al., 2008a, 2008b). The information patients find online increases their ability to select providers and facilities, to compare treatment options, and to learn about complementary and alternative methods of cancer care.

Health information found on the Internet, however, can be confusing. Health issues are complex, and a bump, pain, or ache in one person may have a very different cause and treatment than the same symptom in another person. Healthcare providers go to school for years to learn how to properly diagnose patients' illnesses. A quick look at the Internet can add to a person's knowledge about a symptom or a disease, perhaps allowing someone to recognize and treat a rash caused by poison ivy or to find out when screening colonoscopies are generally recommended for symptom-free adults. More complex issues, however, including symptoms and treatments for cancer, require more complex answers that should be provided by a knowledgeable healthcare professional.

The Internet is a good resource for cancer patients and can be used as part of a patient's overall information gathering and decision making. In fact, recent research indicates that older adults continue to underutilize the Internet and electronic devices when it comes to exchanging of health information

(Saied et al., 2013). So, there is room for improvement in using online resources in cancer care. But the Internet is not a substitute for quality health care and interaction with healthcare providers.

The Internet might be used to find a physician. If someone has just been diagnosed with pancreatic cancer, for instance, that patient might look at the Pancreatic Cancer Action Network website to find information about surgeons and oncologists who have a lot of experience with this relatively rare disease. Healthcare marketing is big business, so individual physicians, hospitals, and diagnostic centers publicize themselves on the Internet and make information easy for prospective and current patients to find. Once the patient has found a physician, that person might use the Internet to get office information and driving directions.

Patients also often search the Internet to verify information they receive from their healthcare providers about their condition and treatment options. Because a cancer diagnosis can be shocking and scary, it is common to seek out additional or confirming information after receiving diagnosis. Some patients will use the Internet also to look up terms used by their provider. What exactly is a *mastectomy*? What does a *radiologist* do? How is *PSA* measured? Answers to all of these basic questions—which may not at first seem basic to the patient—can be found on the Internet.

Using Internet Groups Wisely

The Internet and social media such as Facebook, Twitter, and chat groups offer cancer patients and their families the opportunity to reach out to other people in similar situations, particularly in groups and chat rooms focused on cancer therapy and treatment. Patients can often converse with people who have the same cancer type and stage, who have the same side effects of treatment, or who share similar concerns and fears. A patient or caregiver may feel more comfortable asking embarrassing or difficult questions anonymously or in an online setting. While online information should not substitute for information from a healthcare provider, consider how the following topics might be handled differently in online groups or forums than in typical provider–patient interactions and how each type of interaction—in person or online—might inform decision-making.

- Terminology the healthcare provider uses but the patient doesn't understand.
- Telling friends or coworkers about a diagnosis and treatment.

- How much detail to provide one's children.
- Deciding among treatment options.
- Handling side effects and determining which side effects are normal.
- Where to get supplies like special bras, wigs, hospital beds, and other supplies.
- How to depend on one's family without overburdening them.
- What questions to ask an employer about medical leave from work and how to ensure one is being treated fairly at work.
- Showing gratitude toward healthcare providers, including nurses.
- Local agencies that help with personal care, housecleaning, yardwork, and other tasks.
- Handling emotional stress, moodiness, or depression during cancer care.
- Intimacy and sex life.
- Maintenance after completing treatment.
- Recurrence of a cancer that was treated previously.
- The role of a counselor, minister, or psychiatrist for caregivers.
- Timing FAMLA leave from work when a loved one most needs care.
- Putting one's legal and personal affairs in order after a terminal cancer diagnosis.

Email as Cancer Communication

Email—electronic mail—is an example of computer-mediated communication designed as interpersonal between two (or a few) parties. In some ways, it is like "snail mail" or old-fashioned letter correspondence, with one person making a statement in writing, the recipient reading that statement at some later time, the recipient able to respond in writing, and so forth. Of course, email back-and-forth can happen a lot faster than the postal service can manage. But it is very important to remember that an email conversation is different than a conversation in person in real time. In fact, some people may find email too impersonal to convey information about their cancer care.

That personal distance of email can be a detriment in some situations, but it can be a benefit in other ways. At the beginning of her book *The Middle Place*, Kelly Corrigan (2008) recounts having sent an email message two weeks before her 37th birthday in August to arrange for a lunch celebration. Less than a week later, she was diagnosed with cancer and sent a follow-up message to the same group. She tried to sound brave. She began her message with "Brace yourself. Yesterday, I was diagnosed with breast cancer" (p. 50). She includes a brief overview of her treatment plan—chemotherapy, surgery, radiation—and announces that she'll host a "great party, next summer" (p. 51).

This form of communication allowed Corrigan to communicate her news to friends all at once, instead of one by one. It also allowed her to control the content and tone without being interrupted. Though she admitted to her husband that she was embarrassed by how upbeat she was in the message, email allowed her to present herself as confident and positive about her situation.

In her book *Everybody's Got Something*, Robin Roberts (2014) reminds us that our usual expectations for email correspondence may need to be suspended when it comes to cancer care. Email messages cheered Roberts immensely and were an important source of joy. But her partner, Amber, recounts that it was sometimes difficult to prioritize tasks they intended to do, like respond to email or thank well-wishers for gifts. While support is often welcome, those who call, email, text, or send a gift to someone who is seriously ill should do so with no expectations of immediate reply. Family and friends may expect two-way communication, which isn't always feasible or helpful for the cancer patient and caregivers. Email correspondence may work well when the patient is feeling well, but the side effects of treatment or the progression of the disease can leave a patient without enough energy or clear-headedness to respond quickly or at all. In some situations, caregivers may want to ask a patient whether access to the patient's email account might be shared so that the caregiver can help with responses. Some patients will welcome such assistance, while others will want to maintain privacy and a sense of control by remaining solely responsible for their own email correspondence.

In recent years, message management alternatives have emerged for patients and caregivers. New cancer care related sites such as caringbridge.org are becoming increasingly popular as a hub for message postings as they allow people to easily get updates and offer support and encouragement. Even when using these sites, family and friends should understand that caregivers and patients may be busy and exhausted and may not be up to sending out updates consistently.

An increasing number of healthcare providers are choosing to use email as a way to connect with patients, convey information to their patients and their patients' designated caregivers, and remind patients of appointments and preparation for specific tests. As more people use smart phones, use of text messaging and email will be especially helpful, which allows the recipient to be notified easily when new information is shared and even to sync appointment information to their personal electronic calendars.

When a patient and provider communicate through email, providers should take several important steps to foster ethical and effective communication with patients. Likewise, patients should recognize the benefits and limitations of email communication.

1) Because a patient's medical records are private, the cancer care provider should take necessary steps to authenticate that the person with whom email is being exchanged is the patient or a designated caregiver. Although it seems unlikely, a family member or employer could email a provider for private patient information. The provider should require authentication to ensure privacy. Usually, this authentication is done via a consent form that the patient fills out so that the provider communicates via a secure email address (or phone number) provided by the patient. Some patients may want to avoid listing a work email address or may want to set up a new email account, which can be accessed by both the patient and a designated caregiver, just for healthcare communication. This initial authentication should occur before any online communication with a patient begins.
2) Email correspondence between patients and providers should only occur in existing clinical relationships. Because so much of cancer care is highly personal and individualized, it is essential for any care provider to know a patient's medical history and the specifics of that person's diagnosis and therapy. Email correspondence with online doctors—physicians who have not taken the patient's medical history, seen test results, and examined the individual in person—cannot provide the personalized, accurate, relevant information upon which cancer patients and their families can rely. Although the idea of using technology to anonymously ask questions over the Internet can seem like a time-efficient and cost-saving measure, websites and online services should be reserved for routine or general health questions. Cancer patients need more, including coordinated care from providers who are familiar with the specifics of the case and who will be available for ongoing consultation and care.
3) Providers should give patients clear information in advance about how their time spent in email correspondence will be billed. Often, providers charge fees—usually based on their regular hourly charges—for writing and respond-

ing to email messages from patients. Patients should have a full understanding about whether such fees will be considered allowable expenses based on the healthcare plan under which the patient's health care is covered.

4) Patients and providers should discuss principles for acceptable use of email. It is important to establish in advance a clear understanding of the types of information that should be conveyed through email and circumstances when it would be better to use other communication channels such as face-to-face or telephone conversations. Physicians should present guidelines for email use and make it clear that it's not appropriate for all questions or concerns. In addition, when establishing email ground rules, a patient might ask, "How long should I expect to wait for a reply?" The patient may want to ask for examples of when to use email, perhaps asking which possible side effects should receive immediate attention and, therefore, warrant a phone call or even a trip to the Emergency Room instead of an email message.

Physicians sometimes work long and irregular hours, so when they do have time off, patients can't expect them to answer routine questions quickly if sent via email. Some doctors have what they call *email office hours*. During these designated time periods, patients can expect to receive responses within those hours. Other times, providers may have a version of a 48-hour policy. In that case, providers respond to all messages within a 48-hour or two-day window. If a patient or caregiver needs an immediate answer, email may not be the best way to communicate a question.

Email habits and policies vary from physician to physician, so the important thing is to make sure the expectations for email are outlined and clear to all involved from the get-go to avoid miscommunication. Of course, this occurs not just with email but also with any communication mediated through technology or, in fact, with any communication method at all.

The Cancer Blogosphere and Social Media

Cautions About Sharing Information Online

If you have never blogged or used social media, if you don't readily have at-home access to the Internet, or if you don't feel very well, you may not want to spend your time using online tools to communicate. In addition, many patients don't want to share their stories, either in real time or in hindsight, because they consider health concerns to be private matters. Anyone concerned about privacy should think twice about putting personal information online, even if that information is protected with a strict privacy setting.

Patients who choose not to share information about themselves with many others may want to engage with the blogosphere and social media as readers but not as active participants. Caregivers, too, might find valuable information and encouragement by reading blogs or posts in online communities. Robin Roberts (2014), in her book *Everybody's Got Something*, writes about a blog that she and especially her partner and caregiver read regularly. Her partner found a blog by a man named Scott who was Roberts's age and several months ahead in the same type of treatment. Though they both read the blog, Amber did so more often than Roberts herself. It can be helpful to remember that the patient and the caregiver may share needs and information in different measure and may find different resources useful. While you can't believe everything you read online, Scott's account of his journey made Roberts and Amber feel as if they were following in his footsteps.

While each cancer situation is different, reading what others have experienced can give you a wider context for your situation, sometimes helping you understand that others share your symptoms or concerns, sometimes providing information that can help you form questions for your oncologist. The important thing for anyone to consider is how this sort of computer-mediated communication can foster better cancer care and decision-making for the patient.

Sharing Cancer via Social Media

Some patients may opt for a Facebook page, a Twitter feed, or another social media presence to engage with others beyond reading and information gathering. Facebook encourages brief status updates and sharing links and also allows the user to set a different privacy setting for each post. That way, the patient can share a link to a news story publicly, for example, while sharing a glum mood or next chemo date with friends or even setting some posts for only the patient to read later.

Pinterest and Instagram offer ways that users can share inspirational messages as images. In fact, Shannen Doherty began sharing photographs of her cancer experience on Instagram in 2016. Some cancer research organizations host Google hangouts. Patients can seek the social media option that works for the ways they want to share information.

In addition, Facebook has groups that users create and that other users can join. Patients can ask questions of groups to which they belong, which is called *crowdsourcing* to get opinions and information from a swathe of people. Organizations also often have pages that users can "like" so that they receive information from those organizations in their newsfeeds. Cancer patients can follow the American Cancer Society, for instance, to get regular updates from that organization. Many other social media options, many of which are free, exist for those who want to share and connect with others. Of course, not every patient will find social media a useful part of their communication strategy, and family and friends should be understanding when a patient does not want to use social media to communicate.

Blogging Your Cancer

When Adam Schmitz decided to keep a journal online, he set it up as a private blog on the Caring Bridge website. His family and friends could register at Caring Bridge to create a login and password so that they could read his journal. That way, he could write what he wanted and share it with people he knew without making it public. He could share more personal information, change his mind or his tone of voice, and test out his ideas without worrying that strangers might judge him. He talked there about writing a book about his experience in the future, but he did not want the pressure of making his posts polished or connected to each other while he was undergoing aggressive and demanding treatment.

When we asked Adam's wife, Wooten, whether we could include some excerpts from his private journal in *Conversing with Cancer*, she knew Adam would have thought it a terrific idea. So, an excerpt opens this chapter.

When Patricia Grace King decided to write about her experience with breast cancer, she already had her own website and wanted to make her writing accessible to all, just as she did when she published stories in literary journals. And she wanted to share right away, as her treatment was happening. So, she used a free blogging platform to build her blog as a page on her website. Initially, she committed to posting twice a week—a good rule of thumb for a blog trying to establish a readership—with one post typed up from the handwritten journal she had been keeping and the other exploring some experiences and issues more deeply as short, informal essays. Of course, with the ups and downs of chemotherapy treatment, surgery, and out-of-town appointments and tests, she adjusted her posting schedule as needed.

Amanda Niehaus made yet a different choice when she started her blog. After her experience with breast cancer as a new mother in her thirties, she became especially interested in healthy lifestyle choices and organic food and wanted to use her expertise as a scientist. So she developed a public blog called *Easy Peasy Organic* that includes helpful hints and recipes. Her blog emerged from her experiences with cancer, but she uses it for health advocacy.

Blogging platforms like Wordpress.com are free and relatively simple for users, so technology and social media have changed the options for patients who want to write or talk about their own experiences with cancer. Blogging can be great for self-expression or self-reflection. In fact, you can even set up a blog that only you can access through privacy settings, so that it functions like an old-fashioned diary. As a patient writes a blog, that person may discover thoughts and feelings about illness by putting those thoughts and feelings into words. Blogging can also be great for sharing one's cancer story with others, either as a private blog to which the patient invites readers, perhaps family and friends, or as a public blog from which anyone might gain insight. If a patient likes speaking better than writing, blogs can even be done as video posts—vlogs—or podcasts instead of text posts.

Reading blogs by others or conversing about cancer in online chat groups can help patients understand their situations, make connections with other cancer patients, and ask questions informally. Blogs, online chat groups, and social media like Facebook and Twitter are not substitutes for reliable information from healthcare professionals and organizations, but they do foster communication and community among cancer patients.

Not all cancer patients have access to computers, devices, or wifi, and not all cancer patients will want to use the latest technology for their own healthcare communication. As with many computer-mediated modes of communication, patients will want to consider when and how best to use the technology to make their lives better. Every decision the patient makes about communication should work toward achieving the goal of living the best life possible.

Exercise & Discussion

Technologies have changed nearly every aspect of the way we communicate today. Many of us find information from online searches; we sometimes rely on websites such as WebMD to try to diagnose our latest ailments; and, when the time comes to visit a physician, we supplement what the healthcare provider tells us with information we find online.

1. How can we use existing technologies more effectively to help patients?
2. In what ways can we make sure that all patients are given and get the same information that people with access to the Internet have?
3. How do you think we can work with aging patients who don't use the Internet to help them feel that they are getting the support and additional information they need that younger people might get via the Internet?
4. How might a patient benefit from participation in social media such as Facebook, Twitter, or Instagram? What reasons might an individual have to choose not to have an online presence after a cancer diagnosis or during treatment?
5. Should video chats, online hangouts, and other virtual communities be encouraged as part of typical patient treatment programs?

References

Corrigan, K. (2008). *The middle place*. New York, NY: Hyperion.

Kreps, G. L., Neuhauser, L., Sparks, L., & Villagran, M. (2008a). The power of community-based health communication interventions to promote cancer prevention and control for at-risk populations. *Patient Education and Counseling, 71*, 315–318.

Kreps, G. L., Neuhauser, L., Sparks, L., & Villagran, M. (Eds.). (2008b). Translational community-based health communication interventions to promote cancer prevention and control for vulnerable audiences. [Special Issue] *Patient Education and Counseling, 71*, 315–350.

Roberts, R. (2014). *Everybody's got something*. New York, NY: Grand Central.

Saied, A., Sherry, S. J., Castricone, D. J., Perry, K. M., Katz, S. C., & Somasundar, P. (2013). Age-related trends in utilization of the internet and electronic communication devices for coordination of cancer care in elderly patients. *Journal of Geriatric Oncology*, 5, 185–189. doi:10.1016/j.jgo.2013.11.001

Sparks, L., & Miller-Day, M. (2014). Methodological approaches to eliminating health disparities. In B. Whaley (Ed.), *Research methods in health communication: Principles and Application* (pp. 318–336). New York, NY: Taylor and Francis.

· 11 ·

EXTENDING THE CONVERSATION

A New Theoretical Model for Cancer Communication

before treatment
waiting for blood test results—
I stare at a magazine

in the hallway
before the chemo room
a plate of cookies

accessing my port
the chemo nurse says
don't breathe on it

chemo room—
fluorescent light shining
through infusion bags

four days not seeing
morning sunlight breaking
through the clouds

first day free
from chemo side-effects—
pine needles mulch the lawn

—from "Chemo Room" by Penny Harter

The word cope *comes from the French, meaning to punch with a fist.* Transcend, *a word that comes from Latin through French, suggests an escape from or climbing over of something. Many people with cancer think about their long-term experiences with these concepts—coping and transcending, fighting and surmounting—in mind. Many patients, in the days and years after a cancer diagnosis, articulate new perspectives about themselves and their lives. The word* motto *comes from the Latin meaning* grunt *or* mumble *and has come to refer to a guiding statement of underlying model that encapsulates one's ideals. Cancer can challenge an individual's beliefs, sense of self, and purpose in life in ways that lead to a new understanding or awareness of words by which to live.*

In this chapter, we break new ground by employing the selection, optimization, and compensation model to understand the continuum of cancer care and how providers, patients, and caregivers can create beneficial interactions and make the best decisions possible.

The Selection, Optimization, and Compensation Model and Cancer Communication

The selection, optimization, and compensation (SOC) model was first proposed by Baltes and Baltes in 1990 as a theory of lifespan strategies that create well-being among individuals and has been adapted for many contexts (e.g., Müller, Heiden, Herbig, Poppe, & Angerer, 2015). This model refers to a way to understand how these three strategies of development function over an individual's lifespan to maximize gains and minimize losses. We propose a provider–patient extension of SOC into the context of the cancer care continuum.

As cancer care evolves along a continuum, ranging from prevention, detection, diagnosis, treatment, and survivorship or end-of-life, both patients and providers should consider the SOC model for adapted behaviors. These behaviors are described more specifically in an article by Baltes and Heydens-Gahir (2003). Here, we explain each and then explore them in the context of cancer communication.

Selection

Selection occurs when individuals choose goals for themselves. This process entails allocating resources toward specific outcomes, with the awareness that those resources are limited. The model outlines two kinds of selection: *elective* and *loss-based*. *Elective selection* typically is geared toward increasing function based on existing or potential resources, while *loss-based selection* typically is geared toward maintaining function and is motivated by a lack of an internal or external resource. A person may physically train on a strict schedule—and perhaps spend money on a personal trainer—to build on existing strength and endurance to achieve the goal of completing a marathon. An example of an internal shortcoming that can drive loss-based selection is new loss of vision or another ability that makes achieving some goals more difficult. A lack of insurance coverage could represent a shortcoming in an external resource that could then lead to loss-based choices. Life stage and aging, as earlier application of SOC posited, affect a person's goals, internal and external resources, and selection process. Likewise, cancer or another serious illness affects one's goals, resources, and selection.

Optimization

Optimization occurs when individuals refine their current or available resources to achieve their goals. This process can include practicing new skills, modeling successful behavior, and scheduling time and energy for the optimal achievement of goals (e.g. resting more, more time with family, maintain work hours, etc.). For individuals who are seriously ill, optimization may mean resting more frequently and spending more time with one's family. For others facing a diagnosis such as cancer, optimization could mean maintaining current work hours in order to continue life as usual to the greatest extent possible, thereby optimizing the quality of their current health.

Compensation

Compensation occurs when individuals find alternative methods of achieving goals or maintaining function when faced with diminishing or declining resources. Because health can be considered a resource in this extension of SOC, compensation plays an important role when it comes to a cancer diagnosis, treatment, and progression of illness or recovery. Compensation also occurs when an individual is overloaded and at the limits of resources, including physical or emotional energy. Examples of compensatory strategies include substituting one resource for another, using additional external resources, ignoring unrelated or lower-priority goals, and engaging in psychological therapy or support systems. A patient might sell property to bring in money, put marathon training on hold indefinitely to use physical energy for doctor's appointments, or attend religious services or community support groups to foster a sense of well-being in new ways.

The Selection, Optimization, and Compensation Model has been used to understand older adulthood in relation to the physical and mental changes that are likely to occur after the age of 65. Because cancer at any age also causes physical and mental declines, SOC can be extended to understand the continuum of cancer care and to improve cancer communication between providers and patients. SOC is based on the idea that an individual continues to adapt over the entire lifespan and continues to rebalance a variety of gains and losses as part of that ongoing adaptation. As one's sense of normal changes, SOC strategies question normal and, instead, focus on maintaining and maximizing function.

- Selection prioritizes those functions which are highest and are likely to remain highest; the cancer patient can select for one's strengths.
- Optimization emphasizes making the most of one's existing functions and resources; the cancer patient can optimize what one already has and is likely to retain.
- Compensation encourages making adjustments to maintain quality of life despite declines in health; the cancer patient can compensate by making substitutions when losses occur.

The purpose of our extension of the SOC model to the patient–provider relationship, provides a successful relational framework for both informal and formal providers to actively participate and better understand how to help cancer patients live the best lives possible.

SOC in Cancer Communication

The SOC model lends itself especially well to an application along the cancer care continuum. Throughout the continuum of cancer detection, diagnosis, treatment, and survivorship or end of life (National Cancer Institute, 2016) goals and resources must constantly be reevaluated. Having cancer means that there will always exist some sort of physical, financial, or emotional strain on the individual. The tenets of the selection, optimization, and compensation model can function to foster well-being through the process of cancer care.

In this section, we examine some ways that the facets of SOC may appear in the cancer continuum for patients, providers, and informal caregivers. We also identify what health interventions based on this extended SOC model might entail and suggest how this model can, and should, be tested in future research. Because this communication-based extension of SOC takes a relationship perspective to cancer and lifespan, it is useful for cancer patients, providers, and caregivers to study and use and, importantly, for health communication scholars to research further.

Prevention and Detection

For healthy aging generally and cancer prevention specifically, people can optimize their goals for health by exercising more, smoking and drinking alcohol less, and wearing sunscreen. Such healthful habits are likely most beneficial over long time frames. Because it is impossible to prove the negative or to know whether any particular person will develop cancer, optimizing one's resources for cancer prevention can hedge a person's bets on long-term goals for health.

Early detection offers patients the best chance of surviving cancer. Early detection for certain cancers like lung (Baldwin & Callister, 2016) and breast (Kline & Mattson, 2000) is the best defense against mortality, yet screening for early detection remains underused among certain populations. Assessing risk for particular cancers and cancer screening, therefore, should be a part of the standard adaptation of SOC to normal aging.

As people age, selecting certain goals for health and longevity should include disease prevention and detection behaviors, especially routine screening for some more common cancers and for some individuals at higher than average risk. People tend to adapt this sort of elective selection if they belong to social groups that openly talk about cancer screening because external social norms can be powerful motivation for behavior. Individuals may benefit from awareness of this social-norm driven selection and, therefore, surround themselves with people who value cancer screening. Another way to adapt selection is to evaluate the importance of health and the cost to maintain health in terms of loss. While routine screening and checkups can be costly in the immediate sense, long-term costs can be greater for a patient who faces a disease that could have been detected and treated early on. In addition, the earlier expenditure in screening can minimize potential loss of quality of life.

Immediate costs associated with prevention and detection can be redefined as investment in long-term health goals.

In these ways, both selection mindsets and optimization behaviors may help patients engage in more preventative behaviors and remain healthy before any detection occurs. Moreover, they may increase the chance of early detection of cancer, if it develops, to avoid a more advanced diagnosis and more difficult or riskier treatment further along the cancer continuum.

Providers can aid patients in selection, optimization, and compensation behaviors so that patients maximize resources that lead to prevention and early detection. For example, a general practitioner may want to frame cancer screening such as mammography or colonoscopy as elective, part of the overall routine checkup so that it is conveyed as a social norm. Providers may help patients optimize detection behaviors by explaining benefits of early detection in the context of regular medical examinations, sending reminders for appointments, and helping patients feel more in control over their health. Loss-based selection may not be as effective in encouraging screening. Patients with limited time or resources may have trouble using detection resources, and providers may want to consider how they can support the patient's compensation for these resource constraints on a case-by-case basis. For example, a patient who works during the day may need help finding a location that performs early-morning or evening screening, and a patient without a car may need help finding a screening location near public transportation.

Diagnosis

When cancer is diagnosed, the patient becomes a cancer patient and faces the need to adjust current and future goals. In a study of cancer patients' personal goals, researchers found that cancer patients set fewer goals for themselves after a diagnosis. In this study, the goals that the patients formulated were short term, of lesser importance, and related to physical, rather than social, outcomes (Janse, Ranchor, Smink, Sprangers, & Fleer, 2015). A patient beginning chemotherapy treatment, for instance, may want to plan for reducing workload on the job. The individual may be able to share existing projects, stop accepting new projects or tasks until tolerance to treatment is better understood, or request use of accrued sick leave. Because fatigue is one of the most common side effects of radiation therapy, a patient facing this treatment may want to talk with family ahead of time about how to redistribute household responsibilities and chores. As goals shift, cancer patients can optimize the resources they have available and also to compensate for those resources that diminish, resulting in improved well-being overall.

An informal care provider, usually a family caregiver, takes on many new additional responsibilities after a family member is diagnosed with cancer. For instance, Li et al. (2013) discuss the economic burden taken on by informal caregivers within the first year after their partner's initial diagnosis, noting that, on average, more than $6,000 of their annual spending will be related to caregiving. So, it is our contention that the SOC model is relevant not only for the patients themselves, but also for family members affected by a cancer diagnosis and treatment. To better prepare and achieve health outcome goals, informal caregivers can make or adjust a financial plan that takes into account the diagnosis and the ongoing circumstances. Some informal caregivers, for example, may look for ways to compensate for the unexpected economic burden by reallocating existing economic resources, such as savings, or may seek to optimize resources such paid overtime opportunities at work. Other caregivers may optimize accrued paid vacation days or weigh the benefits of family medical leave.

Treatment

Maintaining well-being by employing these SOC strategies can present specific challenges for patients during the treatment phase of the cancer continuum. In the same study on cancer patients' goal setting by Janse et al. (2015), researchers found that the goal selection process was more difficult for patients with more advanced cancer or complicated cancer treatments. Patients with stomas (surgically created holes in the abdomen for elimination of feces), for example, were less able to attain their goals or to believe in the possibility of attaining those goals (Janse et al., 2015). When patients have more complicated cancer treatments, such as stomas, they may need to adjust their goals on a daily basis in accordance with their daily lifestyle changes (Janse et al., 2015). While the stoma is one example of a medical intervention that affects an individual's goals and selection, all cancer patients are likely to grapple with the ways treatment influences goals, resources, and selection.

As cancer treatment procedures adjust over time, cancer patients will likely benefit from adjusting their goals in order to optimize their current resources, including their physical and emotional energy. Coping well with treatment may also be fostered by using the compensatory strategy, such as substituting low-energy leisure activities for high-energy ones or asking for assistance with errands or basic physical care in this often-changing time of life.

Caregivers, too, can employ SOC during a cancer patient's treatment. In a study on informal caregivers of stroke survivors, researchers found that informal caregivers often felt a loss of control over their lives due to the significant responsibility of caring for the patient (Greenwood, Mackenzie, Cloud, & Wilson, 2010). In order to regain some control over their time and schedules, the informal caregivers reported letting go of some activities they had previously enjoyed, thus optimizing their time (Greenwood et al., 2010). These informal caregivers often compensated for their loss of some personal activities by shifting to other activities that better fit into their schedule (like talking with friends over the phone, rather than in person) or by not adjusting at all (Greenwood et al., 2010). To maintain well-being as an informal caregiver, individuals should understand that goal setting and prioritizing will have to occur to optimize time and resources, but caregivers should also remember to compensate for missed opportunities with healthful activities to relieve stress.

Providers themselves may be called upon for support during treatment, when both patients and caregivers can feel a declining sense of control. Providers should bear this in mind and be prepared for patients and caregivers to question their limitations, down to very small lifestyle changes or restrictions. It may be helpful for providers to suggest changes to optimize health during treatment so that patients have concrete action they can take and to help them regain some control over decision-making. This holds true for compensation as well, and providers may want to also have common compensation suggestions on hand for patients and their informal caregivers. Because of their experience with many patients, providers may be able to observe and share lifestyle alternatives that may occur to one patient but not another.

Some types of chemotherapy, for instance, cause increased sensitivity to cold in the mouth, so the oncologist may want to talk with the patient about the days in which that side effect may be more likely to occur so that the patient can adjust expectations for certain foods and beverages. Neuropathy (hypersensitivity or numbness, often in the hands) can be another side effect of chemotherapy. In this case, a provider may suggest keeping a pair of gloves next to the refrigerator so that the patient can compensate for this physical change. If cancer progresses, guiding patients to substitute new, realistic, or focused goals for previous ones can be helpful. Providers may be even more helpful in guiding patients toward additional external resources, including options for pain relief and psychological support, as such resources become necessary to ensure that each patient lives the best life possible.

Survivorship and End-of-Life

Survivorship and end-of-life are times when patients may be faced with more questions than answers. When treatment ends and a patient is no longer showing any signs of cancer or related symptoms, follow-up physical examinations and medical tests often remain a routine part of the individual's experience of the cancer continuum. Patients who survive cancer may face questions as to their new identity as cancer survivors, and the nature of their relationships with others may change. Furthermore, they may face uncertainties of whether the cancer will return or if they are done dealing with this illness. During *survivorship*, when patients move through treatment into life with cancer management or life without cancer, patients may need to optimize their abilities and compensate for all of these mounting uncertainties by establishing boundaries and identities with friends and family in a way they might have never done before. They may also have to compensate for any lifestyle restrictions while they regain strength from treatments. For some patients, cancer will likely not return, and SOC strategies will allow them to return to goals they had put aside or to set new goals for themselves. For others, cancer will return, and the recurrence or a new diagnosis will be a new experience with new challenges.

Survivorship can be an especially challenging time for informal providers. Of course, survivorship is a time to celebrate successful treatment and the potential of living without cancer as a less significant part of one's life than it once was. For these lucky patients and loved ones, it is a time to rekindle relationships and enjoy health together, but this can also be a time of additional shifts in identity. Miller and Caughlin (2013) explain that couples' identities evolve throughout each phase of the cancer continuum and that both patient and caregiver can experience unknown identity shifts and crises. Having adapted their goals and personal needs to align with the needs and goals of the partner experiencing cancer, both loved ones must adjust to the new normal of living without cancer by reevaluating goals and detaching from the cancer. SOC lends itself as a tool for both patient and caregiver during survivorship.

Of course, some patients will not survive cancer and must gradually adjust to living and conversing with cancer as they come to terms with an undesirable outcome. For patients at the end of their lives, especially older patients, optimizing quality of life is often the most important part of SOC. External motivation may have little effect on priorities or behavior, and loss-based selection may predominate as physical abilities diminish. Optimization and compensation may seem especially limited, yet may be all the more important for the patient's well-being. Small gains and pleasures may have great resonance, and small substitutions may offer great comfort.

SOC lends itself to use by both patient and caregiver at end-of-life. When a loved one dies, the caregiver must engage in selecting new goals for oneself, optimizing those goals, and potentially compensating for all that may have been lost, which is likely to be an incredibly difficult yet important process. A caregiver must go through unknown identity shifts from being a family caregiver to not being one. It may be difficult for the caregiver to pick up where one left off before becoming an informal caregiver, so a new selection process must occur whether one faces the challenges of survivorship or the end of a loved one's life.

Hospice, which we have discussed in other contexts in this book, offers support for adapting selection, optimization, and compensation for end-of-life. Physicians should be prepared to talk with terminally ill cancer patients about the ways that hospice can support a person's changing priorities, help a patient optimize quality of life, and offer ways to compensate when time, as well as health and energy, becomes a more starkly limited resource. As pointed out in the introduction to *Communication at the End of Life* (Nussbaum, Giles, & Worthington, 2015), "Decision making and negotiation regarding the types of care and length of treatment at the end of life are important communication processes because, oftentimes, making decisions about end-of-life care is one of the few things over which the dying person and family members have any control in the midst of terminal illness" (p. 3).

Patient-Centered Communication about SOC

Patient-centered communication should be embedded in health campaigns in each and every patient and provider interaction. Ideally, SOC takes a relational approach to the provider–patient interaction, suggesting that it should be applied and discussed openly between patient and provider in annual physicals as well as across the healthcare continuum after cancer is detected. For that to occur, providers need to be trained in and comfortable talking about ways selection, optimization, and compensation can help their patients live the best lives possible. As part of treatment, providers should reevaluate goals frequently with their patients and should optimize their own skills and abilities as well as help patients optimize their skills and abilities. Providers should be aware that SOC strategies can extend into survivorship and can also help patients and their families face end-of-life difficulties and transitions. The purpose of patient-centered communication about SOC is to create shared meaning between cancer patients and providers so that patients can make the best decisions for their situations and lead the best lives possible.

Now that we have extended SOC to the cancer care continuum, further research is needed into the ways selection, optimization, and compensation can best be adapted to help each patient negotiate cancer detection, diagnosis, treatment, survivorship, and end-of-life on one's own terms for the best possible outcomes for the particular diagnosis and prognosis. The extension of the SOC model to the provider–patient relationship, therefore, holds a potentially successful relational framework for both informal and formal providers to actively participate and better understand how to help cancer patients live the best lives possible.

Exercise & Discussion

Put yourself in the role of the healthcare provider for a patient with cancer.

- What specific adaptations would you recommend to the patient for selection, optimization, and compensation during each phase of the continuum of cancer care—Prevention, Detection, Diagnosis, Treatment, Survivorship, or End-of-Life?
- How would your recommendations change depending on the phase of life, on the stage of cancer, and also on the patient's circumstances?

Consider working pairs to brainstorm and then practice conversations that discuss these adaptations with one person playing the role of the provider and the other playing the role of patient.

References

Baldwin, D., & Callister, M. (2016). What is the optimum screening strategy for the early detection of lung cancer. *Clinical Oncology*, *28*, 672–681. doi:10.1016/j.clon. 2016.08.001.

Baltes, P. B., & Baltes, M. M. (1990). Psychological perspectives on successful aging: The model of selective optimization with compensation. In P. B. Baltes & M. M. Baltes. (Eds.), *Successful aging: Perspectives from the behavioral sciences*, 1–34. New York: Cambridge University Press.

Baltes, B. B., & Heydens-Gahir, H. A. (2003). Reduction of work-family conflict through the use of selection, optimization, and compensation behaviors. *Journal of Applied Psychology*, 88, 1005–1018. doi:10.1037/0021–9010.88.6.1005.

Greenwood, N., Mackenzie, A., Cloud, G., & Wilson, N. (2010). Loss of autonomy, control and independence when caring: A qualitative study of informal caregivers of stroke survivors in the first three months after discharge. *Disability and Rehabilitation*, *32*, 125–133. doi:10.3109/09638280903050069.

Janse, M., Ranchor, A. V., Smink, A., Sprangers, M. A., & Fleer, J. (2015). Changes in cancer patients' personal goals in the first 6 months after diagnosis: The role of illness variables. *Support Cancer Care*, *23*, 1893–1900. doi:10.1007/s00520-014–2545-0.

Kline, K. N., & Mattson, M. (2000). Breast self-examination pamphlets: A content analysis grounded in fear appeal research. *Health Communication*, *12*, 1–21.

Li, C., Zeliadt, S., Hall, I., Smith, J., Ekwueme, D., Moinpour, C., & Ramsey, S. (2013). Burden among partner caregivers of patients diagnosed with localized prostate cancer within 1 year after diagnosis: An economic perspective. *Supportive Care in Cancer*, *21*, 3461–3469.

Miller, L. E., & Caughlin, J. P. (2013). "We're going to be survivors": Couples' identity challenges during and after cancer treatment. *Communication Monographs*, *80*, 63–82.

Müller, A., Heiden, B., Herbig, B., Poppe, F., & Angerer, P. (2015). Improving well-being at work: A randomized controlled intervention based on selection, optimization, and compensation. *Journal of Occupational Health Psychology*, *21*, 169–181. doi:10.1037/a0039676.

National Cancer Institute. (2016). *Cancer control continuum*. Division of Cancer Control & Population Sciences. Retrieved from https://cancercontrol.cancer. gov/od/continuum. html

Nussbaum, J. F., Giles, H., & Worthington, A. (Eds.). (2015). *Communication at the end of life*. New York, NY: Peter Lang.

· 12 ·

EPILOGUE

Mottos Moving Forward

The difference between luminosity and brightness
is the difference between being

and being perceived, between the energy emitted
and the apparent magnitude. O, to be

significant! To have some scope and scale!
—from "The Habits of Light" by Anna Leahy

Perspectives on Coping With and Transcending Cancer

As *Conversing with Cancer* demonstrates, there is no single formula for communication that works for every healthcare provider and every patient. Each individual negotiates prevention, risk, diagnosis, treatment, survivorship, and end-of-life differently.

Kelly Corrigan (2008) realized that she, like any other cancer patient, must be herself, a soldier among soldiers: "I wear the uniform, I show my scars, I nod through the hero talk. Other vets repel me, and then, just as regularly, they fortify me. Among them I am completely real, not a cancer ambassador, not a patient representative, not 'an inspiration'" (p. 245). Corrigan comes to blows with her situation at one moment and climbs into it in the next so that otherness, acceptance, and transcendence become intertwined. Though not an easy fit, she finds companionship in the cancer community.

Cartoonist Miriam Engelberg (2006) made light of the serious subject of cancer: "The thing is, I'm not suited for cancer either. 'With your tendency toward nausea and obsessive fear of death, you show no aptitude for cancer. Perhaps you should consider high school teaching instead'" ("Teaching High School vs. Cancer"). No one chooses cancer, of course, and Engelberg points out that no one is prepared for all the aspects of the disease and treatment that a patient faces. Once diagnosed, the basic fact of having cancer does not go away, and each patient—and each family—copes differently.

Comedian Glida Radner (2009) came to appreciate what initially seemed especially difficult about having cancer, namely the uncertainty about what's next and how all the parts of the experience of cancer fit together: "So now I've learned, the hard way, that some poems don't rhyme, and some stories don't have a clear beginning, middle, and end. [...] Delicious ambiguity" (p. 254). Radner came to uneasy terms with not knowing and even savored it at times as part of her rich life that included but was not limited to cancer.

Playwright Eve Ensler (2013) ultimately described her experience in confident language: "We are the people of the second wind. We, who have been undermined, reduced, and minimized, we know who we are. Let us be taken. Let us turn our pain to power, our victimhood to fire, our self-hatred to action, our self-obsession to service, to fire, to wind" (p. 216). Ensler transformed the negative into the positive. She worked to transcend the situation in which she might otherwise have ended up feeling trapped.

Literary scholar Susan Gubar (2012) wrote at the end of her memoir about cancer, while still undergoing treatment, "So this is, after all, a happy ending, the happiest ending I can now imagine. [...] For surely the mystic gaits of going along in tandem or side by side cure the spirit, blessing even an ingrate like me with a surplus of wonder for which I am and will be eternally thankful" (p. 263). Not cured of her cancer, Gubar transcends it by opening herself to the possibility of wonder of spirit. She has continued treatment and gone on to write another book about reading and writing about cancer.

Continue the Conversation

You have read this book because communicating about cancer matters to you. Maybe you are studying health communication so that you can improve the healthcare system and make a difference in the lives of patients, caregivers, and providers. Maybe you are an oncologist, a nurse, a lab technician, or a social worker who talks with cancer patients regularly as part of your career. Maybe you were diagnosed with cancer yourself, as were Kelly Corrigan, Miriam Engelberg, Gilda Radner, Eve Ensler, and Susan Gubar, whose words articulate a variety of perspectives of a cancer patient over time. Perhaps, you are an informal caregiver or someone close to you is going through cancer treatment. You are an individual who came to this book because of your particular situation.

We cannot know exactly why you sought out *Conversing with Cancer* or how it may influence your conversations going forward, just as no one can predict who will be diagnosed with cancer. In fact, it remains important to keep in mind what George Johnson (2013) writes in *The Cancer Chronicles:*

> With enough information—demographic, geographic, behavioral, dietary—we can narrow the pool of those at risk for certain cancers. In the future genomic and proteomic scans and technologies not yet know may allow the pools to be narrowed further still. But there is only so far we can go. Whether any one person gets cancer or does not will always remain mostly random. (p. 203)

Readers of this book may employ its principles in different ways in different situations over time. For some of us who are not reading it as patients, we may return to it after a future cancer diagnosis of our own.

Of course, it would be helpful to read *Conversing with Cancer* before really needing it, before diagnosis. It would be helpful if everyone understood, before ever entering the healthcare system, how cancer care works and how to improve communication, strengthen coordination, and, by extension, improve decision-making. But a person never fully anticipates a cancer diagnosis, and even those already engaged with cancer care are rarely prepared for all the possibilities—new questions, new information, new obstacles, new technologies, new variations of treatment—that might emerge over time. Because of this, experts in health communication play an important role in the healthcare system, from prevention and risk to diagnosis and treatment.

We would like to assure our readers that cancer will someday be eradicated, that this book and improving communication in cancer care will no longer be relevant in the not-too-far-off future. But, as we all know, that is not likely the case. At best, cancer will continue to evolve into becoming more manageable like many other diseases. In fact, as medicine enables us to live longer, our bodies' cells have more time to become damaged or make the sort of mistakes that eventually result in the running amok of cell division that is cancer. In Christopher Hitchens's (2012) words, "To the dumb question 'Why me?' the cosmos barely bothers to return the reply: Why not?" (p. 6). As Siddhartha Mukherjee (2010) more formally points out, "[Q]uite possibly cancer is *our* normalcy as well, that we are inherently destined to slouch towards a malignant end. Indeed, as the fraction of those affected by cancer creeps inexorably in some nations from one in four to one in three to one in *two*, cancer will, indeed, be the new normal—an inevitability. The question then will not be *if* we will encounter this immortal illness in our lives, but when" (p. 459). This book and the need to improve cancer care communication is likely to become more relevant in years to come, even as treatment options improve.

So, we have done our best in *Conversing with Cancer* to provide readers with overviews and strategies for remaining attentive, active, and agile in cancer care. Because many of us will be affected by cancer, we must strive for ways to empower ourselves and to allow ourselves to lead the best lives possible, no matter the circumstances and decisions we face. We must converse with cancer because it is not going away from this world any time soon. As Kelly Corrigan (2008) asserts about the community she sees among her generation over time and shared experiences, "Because we did all this, in that worst moment, we will transcend" (p. 267). Using *Conversing with Cancer* as a resource, we can handle these necessary conversations in ways that serve us as whole individuals. We can create conversations that can encourage us to transcend, to become fire and wind, to relish ambiguity, to laugh at our shortcomings, and to find our happy endings. It is our fervent hope that health communication scholars and students exposed to this book will use it in their life's work and also share the ideas and best practices with their family and friends who are affected by cancer in some way.

Because we know that there is much more to say and share about cancer and health communication, we invite you to visit the *Conversing with Cancer* website at www.ConversingWithCancer.com. There, you will find links to cancer care resources, additional stories by those affected by cancer, ideas for group discussions and community workshops, and ways to contact us. We have started an important conversation with you, and we want to continue sending you and yours love and light in your life journey.

References

Corrigan, K. (2008). *The middle place*. New York, NY: Hyperion.
Engelberg, M. (2006). *Cancer made me a shallower person: A memoir in comics*. New York, NY: Harper.
Ensler, E. (2013). *In the body of the world*. New York, NY: Metropolitan.
Gubar, S. (2012). *Memoir of a debulked woman*. New York, NY: W.W. Norton.
Hitchens, C. (2012). *Mortality*. New York, NY: Twelve (Hachett).
Johnson, G. (2013). *The cancer chronicles*. New York, NY: Knopf.
Mukherjee, S. (2010). *The emperor of all maladies*. New York, NY: Scribner.
Radner, G. (1989/2009). *It's always something*. New York, NY: Simon & Schuster.

APPENDIX A

Glossary

Scholars in the field health communication will likely be familiar with terms used in this book. *Conversing with Cancer* defines key terms in the text, usually at first use, so that readers less familiar with terminology of health communication studies and cancer care will comprehend as they read. This glossary can be used by readers to locate definitions in the text in order to see terms used contextually for greater comprehension. The glossary may be especially useful for instructors who want to discuss terminology and concepts with students, for students studying health communication, and for providers, caregivers, and patients who want to strengthen their communication by building shared vocabulary.

A

B

C

D

E

F

G

H

I

L

M

N

O

P

R

S

T

APPENDIX B

Suggested Online Resources for Expanded Discussion

While not a comprehensive list, the following online resources about health communication, health literacy, cancer, and cancer care offer ways to extend discussions generally, in relation to specific cancer types, and in connection with each chapter of this book. The authors do not advocate any particular online resource, nor do we advocate using any online resource as a substitute for seeking medical care. In addition, this list is not a comprehensive guide to online resources about cancer. This list will be available and expanded at www.ConversingWithCancer.com.

General

American Cancer Society: http://www.cancer.org
Cancer Care: http://www.cancercare.org
Cancer Financial Assistance Coalition: http://www.cancerfac.org/
Clinical Trials in the United States: http://www.clinicaltrials.gov
Five Wishes: https://agingwithdignity.org/docs/default-source/default-document-library/product-samples/fwsample.pdf
National Cancer Institute (National Institutes of Health): http://www.cancer.gov
People Living with Cancer: http://www.plwc.org

Physician Orders for Life-Sustaining Treatment: http://capolst.org/wp-content/uploads/2015/12/2016_CA_POLST_English.pdf

By Type of Cancer

American Brain Tumor Association: http://www.abta.org
Bladder Cancer Advocacy Network: http://www.bcan.org
Breast Cancer Awareness and Information: http://www.breastcancer.org
Esophageal Cancer Awareness Association: http://www.ecaware.org
Kidney Cancer Association: http://www.kidneycancer.org
Leukemia and Lymphoma Association: http://www.lls.org
Lung Cancer Alliance: http://www.lungcanceralliance.org
Melanoma Research Foundation: http://www.melanoma.org
National Brain Tumor Society: http://www.braintumor.org
National Colorectal Cancer Roundtable: http://nccrt.org
Pancreatic Cancer Action Network: http://www.pancan.org
Prostate Cancer Foundation: http://www.pcf.org
Susan G. Komen (breast cancer): http://ww5.komen.org

Chapter 2

Quick Guide to Health Literacy (US Department of Health and Human Services)
https://health.gov/communication/literacy/quickguide/factsbasic.htm
Culture, Language and Health Literacy (US Health Resources and Services Administration)
https://www.hrsa.gov/culturalcompetence/index.html

Chapter 3

Social Identity and Health: An Intergroup Communication Approach to Cancer (Health Communication; access to full article via library database)
http://www.tandfonline.com/doi/abs/10.1207/S15327027HC1502_3
Cultural Insights: Communicating with Hispanics/Latinos (Centers for Disease Control)

http://www.cdc.gov/healthcommunication/pdf/audience/audienceinsight_culturalinsights.pdf
The Cancer Burden in Latin America
http://www.cancer.org/aboutus/globalhealth/globalinitiativesbyregion/latin-america
Breaking Barriers Between Latinos and Health Care Workers (KFSN-TV)
http://abc30.com/education/breaking-barriers-between-latinos-and-health-care-workers/354195/
Grey's Anatomy, "Bad Blood," Season 9, Episode 13 (ABC)
http://abc.go.com/shows/greys-anatomy/episode-guide/season-9/13-bad-blood

Chapter 4

Self Image and Sexuality (National Cancer Institute)
https://www.cancer.gov/about-cancer/coping/self-image
Cancer Facts & Figures for Hispanics and Latinos (American Cancer Society)
http://www.cancer.org/research/cancerfactsstatistics/hispanics-latinos
Cancer Facts & Figures for African-Americans (American Cancer Society)
http://www.cancer.org/research/cancerfactsstatistics/cancer-facts-figures-for-african-americans
Cultural Diversity and Caregivers (American Psychological Society)
http://www.apa.org/pi/about/publications/caregivers/faq/cultural-diversity.aspx

Chapter 5

Yes, I survived cancer. But that doesn't define me. (TedTalk)
http://www.ted.com/talks/debra_jarvis_yes_i_survived_cancer_but_that_doesn_t_define_me
Talking to Children (National Cancer Institute)
https://www.cancer.gov/about-cancer/coping/adjusting-to-cancer/talk-to-children
Red Band Society (13 episodes, ABC)
http://abc.go.com/shows/red-band-society/episode-guide
The Best Gift I Ever Survived (TedTalk)
https://www.ted.com/talks/stacey_kramer_the_best_gift_i_ever_survived

Chapter 6

Tools for Cross-Cultural Communication and Language Access Can Help Organizations Address Health Literacy and Improve Communication Effectiveness (Centers for Disease Control)
https://www.cdc.gov/healthliteracy/culture.html
Hospice Care (National Hospice and Palliative Care Association)
http://www.nhpco.org/about/hospice-care
Universal Healthcare on the Rise in Latin America
http://www.worldbank.org/en/news/feature/2013/02/14/universal-healthcare-latin-america

Chapter 7

Communication in Cancer Care—Patient Version (National Cancer Institute)
https://www.cancer.gov/about-cancer/coping/adjusting-to-cancer/communication-pdq
Communication in Cancer Care—Health Professional Version (National Cancer Institute)
https://www.cancer.gov/about-cancer/coping/adjusting-to-cancer/communication-hp-pdq
Talking with Your Health Care Team (National Cancer Institute)
https://www.cancer.gov/about-cancer/coping/adjusting-to-cancer/talk-with-doctors

Chapter 8

Changes for the Family (National Cancer Institute)
https://www.cancer.gov/about-cancer/coping/adjusting-to-cancer/changes-for-family
Blessings and Struggles of Caregiving (*Catholic Digest*)
http://www.catholicdigest.com/articles/family/family/2015/10-07/blessings--struggles-of-being-a-caregiver
To the Dying, Spiritual Caregivers Can Be a Godsend (*Boston Globe*)
https://www.bostonglobe.com/metro/regionals/south/2014/04/30/dying-spiritual-caregivers-can-godsend/DnyPQo4X9sIwqHv2JIEeRI/story.html

For Elderly Muslims, Few Care Options Outside Home (*New York Times*)
http://newoldage.blogs.nytimes.com/2011/03/15/for-elderly-muslims-few-care-options-outside-the-home/

Chapter 9

Cancer Treatment and Survivorship (American Cancer Society)
http://www.cancer.org/acs/groups/content/@research/documents/document/acspc-048074.pdf

Chapter 10

Online Communities and Support (American Cancer Society)
http://www.cancer.org/treatment/supportprogramsservices/online communities/

Yale Developing Text System to Remind Breast Cancer Patients to Take Their Medication (Hartford Courant)
http://www.courant.com/health/breast-cancer/hc-breast-cancer-yale-special-text-system-20161001-story.html

INDEX

B

C

D

H

I

J

K

L

M

N

O

P

Q

R

S

T

U

V

W

X

Z

Language as SOCIAL ACTION

Howard Giles
GENERAL EDITOR

This series explores new and exciting advances in the ways in which language both reflects and fashions social reality—and thereby constitutes critical means of social action. As well as these being central foci in face-to-face interactions across different cultures, they also assume significance in the ways that language functions in the mass media, new technologies, organizations, and social institutions. Language as Social Action does not uphold apartheid against any particular methodological and/or ideological position, but, rather, promotes (wherever possible) cross-fertilization of ideas and empirical data across the many, all-too-contrastive, social scientific approaches to language and communication. Contributors to the series will also accord due attention to the historical, political, and economic forces that contextually bound the ways in which language patterns are analyzed, produced, and received. The series will also provide an important platform for theory-driven works that have profound, and often times provocative, implications for social policy.

For further information about the series and submitting manuscripts, please contact:

Howard Giles
Department of Communication
University of California at Santa Barbara
Santa Barbara, CA 93106-4020
HowieGiles@cox.net

To order other books in this series, please contact our Customer Service Department at:

(800) 770-LANG (within the U.S.)
(212) 647-7706 (outside the U.S.)
(212) 647-7707 FAX

Or browse online by series at:

www.peterlang.com

www.ingramcontent.com/pod-product-compliance
Ingram Content Group UK Ltd.
Pitfield, Milton Keynes, MK11 3LW, UK
UKHW021837100926
8556IPUK00004B/389

9 781433 133541